WATERFALL
DIET

THE
WATERFALL
DIET

LOSE UP TO
14 POUNDS
IN 7 DAYS
BY CONTROLLING
WATER RETENTION

LINDA LAZARIDES

piatkus

First published in Great Britain in 1999 by Piatkus Books
This paperback edition published in 2010 by Piatkus
Reprinted 2010 (twice)

Disclaimer: this book is not a substitute for proper medical advice.
All persistent symptoms should be reported to a doctor.

A CIP catalogue record for this book
is available from the British Library.

ISBN 978-0-7499-4253-3

Typeset in Dante by M Rules
Printed and bound in Great Britain by
MPG Books, Bodmin, Cornwall

Papers used by Piatkus are natural, renewable and
recyclable products sourced from well-managed forests and certified
in accordance with the rules of the Forest Stewardship Council.

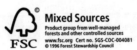

Mixed Sources
Product group from well-managed
forests and other controlled sources
www.fsc.org Cert no. SGS-COC-004081
© 1996 Forest Stewardship Council

Piatkus
An imprint of
Little, Brown Book Group
100 Victoria Embankment
London EC4Y 0DY

An Hachette UK Company
www.hachette.co.uk

www.piatkus.co.uk

Contents

SECTION I: Water Retention: How it starts, its causes, symptoms, research and remedies

SECTION II: The Waterfall Diet

SECTION III: Waterfall Diet Recipes

Acknowledgements

I would like to thank the following people for their help with this book. First, my patients, who showed me what a widespread problem water retention is, and how little it is understood. Second, those doctors and scientists who have found evidence that it is a nutrition-related problem and have tried to tell the world by writing up their work for medical journals. Dr Jean Monro for her ever-generous help and support, Health Interlink Ltd and Great Smokies Laboratory for educating me on liver function, Mr Y. Pang of Payden's chemist, Hailsham, for his assistance with the pharmaceutical section, Carolyn Gibbs for providing many excellent recipes, Dr Judith Casley-Smith and Dr Robert Woodward for information on coumarin, Pennie Hayes for looking after my office, Rita Quinlan of the Nutrition Centre, Heathfield, for assistance with locating health food products, the staff at Piatkus Books and, finally, readers of the previous editions and members of my online forum for helpful comments and suggestions.

How to use this book

There are two types of water retention and at least seven causes. Chapter 1 helps you find out whether you have water retention. Chapters 2–8 help you find out which type and why. In order to fight your particular type of water retention, you will need this information, so there is a short questionnaire at the start of each chapter. Each chapter also has a case history to help you get the picture. The panels of text at the end of the chapters provide more in-depth information and can be skipped if you prefer.

For some people, the cause of water retention is fairly straightforward, like a food allergy or protein deficiency. Once you eliminate the foods that are piling on the water weight, you can lose a lot of weight very quickly – up to 14 pounds in the first week. This weight loss is quite safe. As long as you are drinking enough fluids you don't need to worry about becoming dehydrated or about losing weight too quickly.

Some people only lose a couple of pounds of water weight at first. This may be far from your target, but is still important. Water retention cools down your metabolism and makes it harder to burn body fat. So the Waterfall Diet can also help other diets to work better.

Chapters 9 and 10 will be of special interest to you if your water retention is mainly in your tummy or your legs. Chapters 1–10 mention many foods, nutrients and herbal medicines which help to combat nutritional therapy. Chapter 11 gives more information about these remedies and also covers others which have not yet been discussed. It is intended as a useful reference.

After reading Chapters 1–11, you are ready to start the diet, which aims to put right what has caused your water retention.

The Waterfall Diet itself is in three parts. Phase I aims to shed excess fluid as quickly as possible. Phase II is for finding out what foods are safe to eat without bringing a return of your water retention. Phase III is more long term and is different for everyone. You will know what to eat in Phase III once you have completed Phases I and II.

The Waterfall Diet is not a low-calorie diet. If you have been used to starving yourself you will find it a great relief, although you may miss some of your favourite foods during Phases I and II. Phase III is much easier and aims to prevent your water retention from returning.

Water retention or fluid retention?

Most people use the term 'water retention', but strictly speaking, 'fluid retention' is more correct, as the fluid retained in your tissues is not pure water.

Note for doctors and dieticians

As medicine becomes more and more specialised, it is inevitable that the 'big picture' represented by the enormously complex human body must become more and more elusive. But without seeing more of the big picture, it is difficult to give patients what they really want: to be well again. Instead, medicine is resorting to superficial palliatives: painkillers, anti-inflammatories, steroid creams and antidepressants, and the removal of body parts if they become too painful or dysfunctional. Chronic diseases, ailments and disabilities are now damaging the lives of about one third of the UK population.

This book approaches a very common and distressing medical problem – idiopathic oedema – by using a synthesis of knowledge from many disciplines, including lymphology, immunology and endocrinology. It demonstrates that trying to see more of the big picture can open up a whole new world to the health practitioner – a world where symptoms and lifestyle become clues and the doctor becomes a detective tracking down causes of ill health. While explained in terms simple enough for the lay person to understand, this book is nevertheless full of medical information based on research published in peer-review journals.

Most of your patients will welcome this highly practical treatment protocol for obesity that does not respond to calorie-controlled diets or to the treatment of recognised metabolic disorders. If you email your credentials to waterfall2000@health-diets.net, I will be glad to supply non-profit or National Health clinics and health centres with a single condensed information and diet sheet which can be photocopied for your patients' use. In return, I will ask you to send me the results of any clinical audits from the use of the Waterfall Diet in the treatment of obesity or idiopathic oedema.

Linda Lazarides

SECTION I

Water Retention:
How it starts, its causes, symptoms, research and remedies

CHAPTER 1

Could water retention be your problem?

To be able to sit on the lavatory and urinate away up to 20 lb of excess body weight in a few days probably sounds like something out of your wildest dreams. Yet many people have achieved this and are delighted with the results. Right now, scientists all over the world are looking at the causes of water retention and helping us to understand how it can affect our body weight.

Water retention is a huge problem and it's very difficult to tell the difference between water weight and genuine overweight. If you can answer yes to two or more of the following questions, it is very likely that you could be carrying too much water. Then, by using the advice in this book, you too may be able to urinate some of your body weight away – permanently.

Water retention questionnaire

- Do you eat next to nothing and get plenty of exercise, yet cannot get below a certain weight?
- Press the end of a blunt pencil firmly into your thumb-pad. Does it stay deeply dented for more than a second or two?
- Press the tip of your finger into the inside of your shinbone. Can your finger make a dent?

- Do your legs or ankles ever swell up?
- Does your shoe size seem to increase as you get older?
- Do your rings sometimes seem not to fit you any more?
- Is your tummy often tight and swollen?
- If you are a woman, do you often suffer from breast tenderness?
- Does your weight ever fluctuate by several pounds within the space of only twenty-four hours?

Why fat loss diets may fail

At present most slimming experts have little to offer us other than 'fat loss' diets. These diets assume that all our excess weight is body fat and purely depends on how many calories we consume and how many we burn off as exercise. Yet the human body is far more complex than this. For instance:

- How fast or slow is your metabolism?
- What part do hormones play?

Whatever your particular answer, you will still get the same recommendation: 'Eat fewer calories and exercise more.' The attitude that 'it just takes a little bit of effort' makes people with a weight problem very angry when they have worked hard at dieting and got nowhere. Dozens have consulted me on the verge of tears, torn between feeling desperately guilty that they just couldn't eat any less, and feeling extremely angry that their doctor or dietician would not believe how few calories they were eating. 'My doctor more or less accused me of stuffing myself with chocolate bars and just not admitting it' is a comment I have heard over and over again.

If you have this problem, you already know how frustrating it is to spend a fortune on the gym, to feel constantly depressed from eating a very low-calorie diet without any of your favourite foods, to get up early to go running before work – and then to be accused of lying because you still haven't reached your target weight. It is not unusual for some people actually to gain weight when given a calorie-controlled diet, because they had previously been eating only 500–800 calories a day. Again, it is hard to make anyone believe this.

If this sounds like you, your problem is not related to calories! Body fat is a form of stored energy. As we know, energy is measured in calories: when we say that a certain amount of a food provides us with one calorie, we mean that this food can yield enough energy to raise the temperature of one gram of water by one degree Celsius. One kcal or Calorie (with a capital C) is equal to 1,000 calories.

Calories that we have absorbed from our food, but which remain unused because our level of physical activity is too low, go into storage as body fat. So if we reduce our calorie intake enough so that our normal level of physical activity burns up all the calories we eat, plus some of the calories that we have stored away as fat, we will start losing fat. If at the same time, we increase our physical activity by exercising, stored fat will be lost even more quickly. So by all the laws of science, it stands to reason that, if a calorie-controlled diet is only partly effective, it is not your body fat that is making you overweight.

Hormone imbalance

Sometimes, of course, your hormones are to blame. For instance, a thyroid deficiency will make your metabolism slow down. Your body fat accumulates more easily and burns off more slowly. But your doctor will normally be able to rule out a problem like this with a test and give you thyroid hormone supplements if necessary.

The role of water

One thing which is very rarely taken into account when you are given a weight-loss programme is water. Did you know that your body actually consists of 50–60 per cent water?

Water is found both inside and outside our cells. It forms part of our blood, helping to carry our blood cells around the body and keeping important nutrients in solution so that they can be taken up by tissues such as glands, bone and muscle. Even our organs and muscles are mostly water.

Your body uses a complex system of hormones and hormone-like substances called prostaglandins to keep its volume of fluid at a constant level. So if one day you drink a lot more water or other fluid than usual, you will not end up weighing more; your kidneys will quickly excrete the excess as urine. Likewise, if you do not get enough to drink, your body will hold on to its precious fluids and you will urinate much less than usual.

But what if this system goes wrong and fluid accumulates instead of being excreted? If you have no particular medical symptoms, the chances are that mild water retention, amounting to, say, 7–20 lb of body weight, would not be recognised as fluid. You or your doctor would simply believe that you were overweight due to eating too much or not exercising enough.

How and where does fluid accumulate?

If you have great difficulty in reaching a normal weight and if your doctor cannot find any medical explanation, the chances are that your fluid balance mechanisms have gone wrong and you are not excreting enough water. Water retention means that instead of consisting of 50–60 per cent water, your body weight may be 65 per cent water or even more.

Water retention is said to result from changes in the pressure inside your tiniest blood vessels (capillaries) or changes that make them too leaky. Fluid rich with oxygen and vitamins passes from your capillaries into the surrounding tissues, where it nourishes your cells and eventually returns to the capillary. But if the pressure is wrong, or the capillaries are too leaky, then too much fluid accumulates in the 'tissue spaces' between the cells and cannot get back again.

Water retention can be very hard for a doctor to diagnose. Almost all your body's tissues have plenty of capacity to hold a little more water without looking abnormal. For example, excess fluid could be making your tummy look rather large. When you pinch it, you can feel its normal covering of fat. You may easily believe that your tummy's size is due to this fat. But if you lose your excess fluid your tummy may subside and flatten, so that you can see you have no more fat there than on the rest of your body. Of course, a tummy with slack, poorly toned muscles due to lack of exercise can also look big. Good muscle tone is very important for maintaining a good figure.

Types of water retention

Swollen legs and ankles or a very swollen tummy can be caused by liver, heart or kidney problems. Doctors call this 'oedema' and in these cases there is often too much water in the blood as well as in the tissues. But there is also a 'Type II' water retention which is mostly due to reversible problems such as vitamin or mineral deficiencies and over-production of histamine. In Type II water retention there is too much water in the tissues but sometimes not enough water in the blood.

Could you be retaining water?

How will you know if your fluid balance has gone wrong? It can be hard to tell if your excess weight is mostly water, since water is everywhere in the body. Even your doctor will have difficulty confirming whether you are retaining fluid. Doctors can tell if you have the severe form of water retention known as oedema by pressing a fingertip into your shinbone. If it leaves a dent, you are definitely retaining a great deal of water. Swollen feet or ankles can also be a sign, since excess fluid often collects in the lower half of the body. Sometimes the tummy will be tight and swollen (as in premenstrual water retention) or the face puffy. However, you can have water retention without exhibiting any of these signs. On the other hand, rapid weight fluctuations, where you notice from time to time that you suddenly weigh several pounds more (or less) than you did twenty-four hours ago are a sure sign of water retention; only water can cause such a rapid change in your weight.

Dos and don'ts

If you believe that you suffer from water retention, don't be tempted to drink less. You must drink enough to allow your kidneys to flush the daily waste products out of your bloodstream. If not, your water retention won't improve – it may even get worse. And with Type II water retention your blood can actually become dehydrated if your fluid intake is too low.

The best drink is plain water. The worst drinks are tea, coffee and alcohol, which have a diuretic effect. A diuretic is something which stimulates the kidneys to drain fluid from the blood, but this is not always desirable. If you have Type II water retention, diuretic drinks can even make it worse. Diuretic medicines and herbal products should also be treated with caution.

Alcohol particularly dehydrates you. It reduces the effectiveness of anti-diuretic hormone (ADH), a hormone which slows down your urine production when your blood fluid levels are getting low. Drinking a pint of water before going to bed after you have consumed a lot of alcohol can help to reduce both the dehydration and the hangover which results from it!

As with all health matters, the solution to your water retention will depend on the cause. This book describes all the known causes. Once you know why you have water retention you will often be able to put right the harmful changes in your body which have led to it, using the simple dietary measures described in Section II. Then you will literally be able to urinate away much of your excess body weight, sometimes within just a few days.

Some facts about water

Water is the most abundant substance in your body, found inside and around each of your cells and in your bloodstream and vital fluids. Water is vital to your body. In a temperate climate, adults can live for up to ten days without water and children for five days. Because your body could be severely damaged by losing only ten per cent of its normal water levels, your body tries to keep its water balance as even as possible by making you feel thirsty when it is beginning to get dehydrated. Signs of dehydration include lethargy, nausea (including the morning sickness of pregnancy), heartburn, indigestion, constipation, dry skin and inflammation. Dehydration shrinks the cartilage in your joints, making them more susceptible to friction and arthritis. In fact, chiropractors sometimes cure back pain and painful joints by asking people to drink water instead of tea and coffee.

Water is an essential component of all your body's living cells. Also, by being dissolved in water, many important vitamins, minerals and other vital substances, as well as waste products produced by your cells, can be transported to where they are needed in your body, or to sites of processing and excretion. Water also helps to regulate your body temperature by producing sweat when you get too hot. The evaporation of sweat has a cooling effect on your skin.

Other uses of water by your body include the production of saliva, which helps you to chew your food, and the production of digestive juices. Between 12 and 15 pints (7–8.5 litres) of water a day are extracted from the fluid in your tissues to make these juices. After digestion the water is reabsorbed and returned to your tissues. Contrary to popular belief, you do not need to drink fluid with your meals to 'wash down' your food – it is better if you do not dilute your digestive juices too much.

Water does not just come from the liquids you drink. Up to 2 pints (1 litre) a day can come from food. Fruit, salads and vegetables may contain up to 95 per cent water. Even meat is about 50 per cent water and fish about 70 per cent water after cooking. Bread and cheese contain 35 and 40 per cent water respectively. Try leaving them to dry out and see how much they shrink. Even dried fruit is still 20 per cent water.

More than ¼ pint of water every day is actually manufactured by your body. Known as metabolic water, this is formed when food is converted into energy. Your body produces nearly a tablespoon of water from every 100 calories of food you consume. This water can even be produced from completely dry food; it has nothing to do with the water content of the food itself.

How much water do you need?
Water is lost from your body in urine, sweat, stools and as water vapour in your breath. Heavy sweating can amount to several pints of water a day. Water losses through your breath probably amount to about half a pint a day in normal conditions.

Most of your water is lost through urine, and it is essential to drink enough fluid to produce the amount of urine that your kidneys need to flush out waste products. If your urine looks very concentrated, you are probably not drinking enough. Scientists estimate that most of us need to drink at least 4–5 pints (2–3 litres) a day – more if water losses have been high, for instance if you are breastfeeding, or suffer from heavy periods, or diarrhoea, or tend to sweat heavily. It is advisable to drink this amount of fluid even if your thirst levels don't seem to require it. Thirst sensations only begin once dehydration has started. Elderly people in particular often fail to feel thirsty until they are quite dehydrated. Scientific research now shows that drinking more than 5 pints (2.5 litres) of water a day halves your risk of getting bladder cancer.

The best drink of all is plain water. Drink it on its own or use it to dilute drinks like soup and fruit juice. A mixture of sparkling water and fresh fruit juice is much better for you than canned fizzy drinks, which are often high in sodium, sugar and chemicals. It tastes good too. Weak fruit or herb teas, such as rosehip, blackcurrant, fennel or chamomile – preferably without sugar, are also good choices, and can be drunk hot or cold.

Low-calorie diets and false weight loss

Water amounting to several pounds of body weight is always lost in the early stages of a low-calorie diet. You urinate this water away within two days when your body uses up its stored carbohydrate, found in muscles and the liver. These carbs are bound up with three times their weight in water, and when the carbs go, the water goes too. The problem is that as soon as you start eating normally again, your body puts carbs back into storage and the water comes back too. This effect is responsible for much yo-yo dieting, since dieters believe that they have lost true body weight when they have not. If you have ever tried a short low-calorie diet you probably know how disappointing it is to regain those lost pounds as soon as you resume a normal calorie intake. The Waterfall Diet differs as it helps you to reduce water weight and keep it off.

CHAPTER 2

Allergic water retention:
How your favourite foods could
be turning you into a sponge

One of the biggest causes of water retention is food allergy, a problem which could mean that you start holding on to water like a sponge after eating certain foods. If you eat those foods several times every day, your body will never get the chance to release this excess fluid. This chapter explains what allergies can do and how they can develop due to a condition known as 'leaky gut syndrome'.

Case report: Marjorie lost nearly 14 lbs in one week

Marjorie was a 48-year-old supervisor of a care home for the elderly. Although she ate a strict calorie-controlled diet and was on her feet from 7 a.m. until 9 p.m. most days of the week, up and down stairs, her weight would not budge from 12 stone (168 lb). Worst of all, it was creeping slowly upwards, despite the fact that for the last four years she had eaten little but salad with a small portion of lean grilled meat or fish, and thin wheat crackers.

To find some clues as to what might be causing the problem, I asked Marjorie if she ever suffered from any niggling ailments. It turned out that her doctor had diagnosed arthritis because she had a constant pain in her knees, made much worse by walking upstairs. She had to take painkillers every day.

When I looked at Marjorie's knees, they appeared quite swollen. I was fairly sure that she did not have arthritis but a food allergy which was swelling her up with fluid and making her knees feel tight and painful. I put her on the Waterfall Diet.

After a few days, I got an excited phone call. 'I just can't seem to get off the loo,' she told me, 'I've been producing buckets and buckets of urine and my clothes are so loose they're hanging off me!'

Marjorie lost nearly 14 lb in that first week. Two weeks later, when she saw me again, she was ecstatic: 'I've been constantly on the loo again and have lost another 7 lb. My knee pains have completely gone and I'm feeling so full of energy for the first time in years that I'm going to start an exercise class next week!'

Marjorie lost a total of 22 lb on Phase I of the Waterfall Diet, and to tell the truth it was extremely hard for me to get her off it. She was buying new clothes since her old ones didn't fit her any more, toning up her body with exercises and starting to take care of her appearance again. Within a few months she was looking ten years younger.

Food allergy and leaky gut questionnaire

- Does your weight sometimes go up or down by 3 lb or more in a single day?
- Has your doctor ever diagnosed you as allergic, even when you were a baby?
- Do you suffer regularly from headaches or migraine?
- Do your fingers or knees regularly feel puffy or painful?
- Do you feel slightly congested in your nose or sinuses a lot of the time, or suffer from asthma or hay fever or a lot of mucus?

- Do you regularly suffer from bloating and flatulence (especially after eating) or diarrhoea?
- Do you sometimes suffer from eczema or other skin rashes?
- Have you ever been diagnosed with irritable bowel syndrome?

If you have answered 'yes' to two or more of these questions, there is a strong likelihood that you are a food allergy sufferer. If you have answered 'yes' to question 1, your weight problem is probably due to allergic water retention.

How can food make you retain fluid?

As yet, most doctors are reluctant to believe that food affects people in this way, but some medical researchers have made a special study of it. One French kidney specialist, Dr G. Lagrue from the Henri Mondor Hospital in Créteil, France, has observed that quite frequently a straightforward case of food allergy is mistaken for the serious kidney condition known as nephrotic syndrome, which results in severe water retention due to kidney failure. It appears from his research that some people can react so badly to certain foods that their kidneys behave as if they have this disease.

Patients whom Dr Lagrue has encountered with this kind of food sensitivity have recovered from what was originally diagnosed as nephrotic syndrome after avoiding foods such as cow's milk, pork, wheat, beef and egg. He has found that most of these patients are allergic to several foods and that the problem foods vary from person to person.

It looks very much as though Marjorie's water retention, and that of people similar to her, was a very mild form of the type of allergy that Dr Lagrue describes. In her case, the problem foods turned out to be wheat and yeast. These foods were sending Marjorie's body systems haywire and hindering her blood vessels and kidneys from doing their normal job of siphoning off excess fluid from her tissues.

Water retention is probably the most common symptom of food allergy that I have come across.

What causes food allergies?

In Marjorie's case, her problems only started when she was in her forties. She had never had much of a weight problem until then, no pains in her knees and no fatigue. A lot of people have told me they don't understand how a food allergy (or intolerance, as it is more correctly termed) can start apparently out of the blue like this, but the explanation is straightforward. Most experts in food intolerance are now agreed that it is caused by a damaged intestine leaking undigested food particles into the blood circulation. The particles – which should not be in your blood – set off immune system reactions which subsequently cause your symptoms. The kind of damage which leads to this problem is caused by constant irritation of the intestinal lining.

What can irritate your intestines?

As we grow older, our digestive juices tend to get weaker. Our stomachs can become much less efficient at producing acid; in fact, up to 40 per cent of elderly people are thought to have insufficient stomach acid when digesting a meal. Good acidity levels are needed to start off the rest of the digestive process, so it is easy to see how some people could end up with quite a lot of partly undigested food in their lower intestines. Only the upper part of the intestines is designed to come into contact with undigested food. Lower down, it causes irritation and inflammation. You can't necessarily see the undigested particles in your stools. Digestion has to be very poor indeed before your stools start to look abnormal.

Your body cannot use food until it has been reduced to its smallest possible particles, known as sugars, amino acids and fatty acids. The lining of your intestine normally allows only these items (plus water and other desirable substances) to pass through it into your

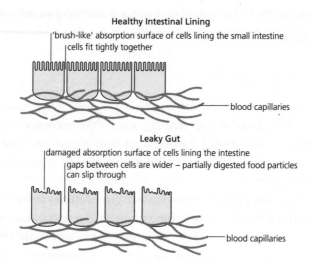

How the intestinal lining becomes 'leaky'

blood circulation. But when your intestine gets irritated and inflamed, it produces histamine, which makes it porous, so it starts to leak bacterial toxins and undigested food particles into your bloodstream. Your blood can carry these particles all around your body.

In your blood, your immune system locks on to the particles and treats them like 'foreign invaders'. So food allergy symptoms can be very similar to those caused when your immune system is attacking invading bacteria:

rashes
swellings
joint pains
headaches
mucus
stuffy nose
fatigue
flu-like sensations
diarrhoea

If you suffer from allergy-related water retention you will probably, like Marjorie, have one or more of these other symptoms too.

The stress connection

Some people only become allergic to a food after a period of great
stress in their lives. Stress can play havoc with your digestion, and
so the vicious circle begins: poor digestion > gut becomes inflamed
and leaky > undigested particles get into blood circulation >
immune system reacts to them, producing allergic symptoms and
water retention.

It is a vicious circle because if your gut becomes inflamed, its
delicate mechanisms for absorbing properly digested food can also
start to malfunction. Mild nutritional deficiencies can develop as
some of your food passes straight through you without being
absorbed. Partly undigested carbohydrates can be seized by
hungry bacteria which reside in the lower part of your gut. These
are the 'undesirable' bacteria which, even though they don't cause
diseases, produce irritating toxins so need to be kept under control. If they thrive too much, these bacteria gradually extend
upwards, colonising your small intestine. Their presence there
causes even more inflammation.

In the early part of the twentieth century, natural medicine
practitioners regularly used to recommend fasting as a cure for
health problems. We know now that fasting regimes probably
worked because, by emptying the digestive system for a while,
they could starve the undesirable bacteria and so help to break the
vicious circle described here.

Which foods cause allergies?

If you have a food intolerance, this will probably involve a food
which you eat very often, such as wheat (from bread, pasta, flour,
cakes, biscuits and so on), eggs or dairy produce. These three
foods are quite hard to digest. If you are allergic to shellfish, for

instance, you would usually know it because most people do not eat shellfish every day – it is easy to associate the symptoms with the food. But if you are allergic to a food that you do eat every day, perhaps only in tiny amounts like egg in a cake or in ice cream or pancakes, your symptoms will either be present more or less all the time or will come and go at random, never allowing you the chance to make the association.

One woman I treated suffered from migraine only when she was under stress. Yet once she was on the Waterfall Diet she never got migraine again, even when she was under a great deal of stress. For her, the Waterfall Diet had revealed an allergy to milk and other dairy products, and by steering clear of these foods she was able to remain symptom-free.

Multiple allergies

Sometimes an allergy sufferer will eventually start reacting to many different foods. This is known as 'multiple allergy syndrome' and is a sign of considerable damage to the intestinal lining and probably also liver stress. The damaged intestinal lining will be allowing many toxins, such as those produced by intestinal bacteria, to pass through it into the bloodstream. The liver, which has to process toxins, then has a greatly increased workload and its enzymes can become overloaded. When this happens, the allergy sufferer can start to feel unwell not just after eating, but also after breathing fumes such as vehicle exhaust fumes or artificial perfumes and air fresheners.

Dr Lagrue reports that most of his patients suffering from allergy-related kidney malfunction and the resulting severe water retention have multiple allergies, including both foods and fumes.

Antibiotics

People who have taken a lot of antibiotics often suffer more from undesirable intestinal bacteria. Your intestines provide a home to many species of bacteria and yeasts or fungi. Some of these bacteria produce very irritating toxins and acids, and are normally kept under control by the other, more 'friendly' bacteria such as Acidophilus (as found in yoghurt). But when you take antibiotics, the friendly bacteria are killed and can no longer do this job. They do eventually re-establish themselves, but if you have been treated with antibiotics for some time, their recovery could be a long process.

The following type of case is very common, and if it sounds like you, you might, in addition to the Waterfall Diet, be in need of treatment to help re-establish your friendly gut bacteria. This would help to heal your leaky gut and prevent you from developing more allergies.

Case report: John regained his energy

John suffered badly from acne and eventually his doctor prescribed antibiotic treatment which lasted about six months. After two months, John noticed that he suffered more from intestinal gas and occasional bloating than he used to, but thought little about it. These, however, were signs that his intestines were not absorbing food properly and were becoming inflamed.

A year later, John was beginning to develop sinus problems and often seemed to have a stuffy nose and excess mucus. He felt bloated most of the time. He was also finding it hard to get up in the mornings – a problem he had never experienced before. He would sometimes fall asleep in the afternoon at weekends. Although only thirty-five, he put it down to simply getting older. He did not worry much until he found himself sleeping ten hours a night and still waking unrefreshed. When his doctor told him there was 'nothing wrong' with him, he consulted an alternative doctor who specialised in chronic fatigue syndrome.

The new doctor had John's urine tested and found large

amounts of a substance that only occurs in the human body when it has a fungus infection in the intestines. John was put on a special diet, plus herbs and supplements to control the fungus and help heal his intestinal wall. He quickly lost his sinus problem, which only occurred when he ate dairy products, and over the next six months he gradually regained his energy levels. His tiredness had been caused by toxins from the fungus leaking from his gut into his bloodstream.

Phase I of the Waterfall Diet is designed to cut out all the foods most likely to be giving you allergic water retention. If you lose a lot of weight very quickly during Phase I, it is very likely that your problem is allergy-related. Phase II allows you to test yourself for food allergies so that you will know which foods bring on your problem and you can avoid those foods when you move on to Phase III. To receive treatment for a leaky gut, you will need to consult a nutritional therapist or naturopathic nutritionist (*see Useful Addresses on p.276*).

The chemistry of allergies

Doctors who specialise in nutritional therapy believe that up to one-third of the Western population suffers from food allergy – the developing of symptoms after consuming certain foods. Symptoms are related not to the substance eaten, but to our reaction to it. So any food can cause any of a hundred symptoms. Wheat might cause headaches or irritable bowel syndrome for some people, dairy products or eggs could produce them in others, or maybe produce skin rashes or asthma attacks instead. There are two types of allergy: classical allergy and intolerance or sensitivity reactions.

Classical allergy

This type shows symptoms rapidly and usually produces a rash when the skin is pricked with the offending substance (this is known as a skin prick test). Hay fever, coeliac disease (diarrhoea after eating flour or cereals) and asthma attacks induced by contact with animal fur or house dust mites are all classical allergies. Anaphylactic shock, where the blood pressure falls to life-threateningly low levels, is also a classical allergic reaction, and can cause death. When people die after eating peanuts, for example, it is as a result of anaphylactic shock.

Intolerance or sensitivity reactions

Here, symptoms are often delayed, intermittent or chronic (long term), and although histamine may be produced, a skin prick test does not usually cause a rash because a different type of immune system reaction is involved. Instead of classical allergy symptoms, food intolerance reactions are more likely to cause symptoms such as migraine, irritable bowel syndrome, joint pains, chronic fatigue and water retention.

As explained previously, food intolerance reactions are thought to be due to a combination of incomplete digestion and a leaky intestinal lining (*see p.15*). When partly digested proteins, known as peptides, escape through the leaky gut into the blood circulation, the immune system attaches proteins known as IgG antibodies to them. When these clumps of peptide and antibody (known as circulating immune complexes) come into contact with white blood cells, they stimulate them to release histamine.

Histamine and water retention

Histamine is a chemical responsible for the physical symptoms experienced by allergy sufferers. If you have ever suffered from hay fever or insect bites, you will be familiar with some of its effects. Histamine dilates your blood capillaries, making them leak extra fluid into the area. This fluid carries white blood cells to the tissues so that the 'invaders' can quickly be dealt with. It also creates swelling and sometimes redness and itching. If histamine is released several times every day, the tissues may never have a chance to release this fluid. Sometimes a few hours' fasting (e.g. overnight) may result in fluid loss, so if you find that you have to get up most nights to urinate and that you weigh several pounds less in the morning, this could be the reason.

Allergy testing

If a doctor suspects the presence of an allergy, he or she will normally use skin prick tests and patch tests, where the test substance is placed in contact with your skin. These tests are good for substances like pollen which react with your skin or nasal passages, but are not suitable for food intolerances. Commercial laboratories sometimes offer blood tests, in which allergies are identified by seeing how your blood cells react when brought into contact with certain foods. This can be unreliable, since, in your body, food would never normally come into contact with your blood.

The Waterfall Diet provides a highly accurate testing method for food intolerances. In technical jargon, it is known as the 'avoidance and challenge' method. More than nine out of ten food allergy sufferers will be able to identify their problem foods if they follow the instructions carefully.

If you believe you have multiple allergies, you should consult a nutritional therapist or a doctor specialising in nutritional therapy (*see Useful Addresses on p.276*). These specialists will help you to improve your digestive ability and repair the damage caused by intestinal inflammation.

CHAPTER 3

Are you getting enough protein?: Protein helps you release excess fluid

A lack of protein in your diet can cause water retention. We have all seen pictures of developing world children with big bellies swollen by water retention and matchstick arms and legs. The technical name for their condition is 'protein-energy malnutrition' and means that they are not consuming enough protein or enough calorie-rich foods in general. The lack of protein in these children's diets prevents their liver from making enough of a substance called albumin, which is essential to prevent water retention.

It seems impossible that in the affluent West anyone could suffer from protein deficiency. In fact most books on nutrition warn us that we are probably eating too much protein and should concentrate more on fruit and vegetables. But some people take this too literally.

Case report: Lesley only lost weight by eating more calories

Lesley, a young advertising trainee working in London, had been fighting a weight problem since her teens. Although then she was no more than about a stone (14 lb) overweight, she felt fat and ugly, especially on the sports field, where she really wanted to shine but had little confidence due to her weight. At fifteen, after trying various diets without much success, she managed with a great effort of willpower to lose 18 lb by following a diet of just fruit and vegetables and a little dry toast. Soon afterwards she decided to stay on a vegan diet (vegans abstain completely from eggs, dairy produce and fish as well as meat), because she did not miss meat and dairy products and felt that this kind of diet was kinder to animals.

Lesley felt great with her new figure and, having lost so much weight, she felt that she could relax her calorie intake and began eating chocolate, potato chips and other sugary, fatty foods again. But once she started she could not stop and the weight problem came back with a vengeance. By seventeen, Lesley weighed more than ever. She was a typical 'yo-yo' dieter, alternating between starving herself for a few weeks and then bingeing on chocolate when the weight had come down a few pounds.

Finally, the scales refused to budge any further, even when Lesley was eating well under 1,000 calories a day. When she consulted me, the first thing I noticed was how low in protein her diet was. She ate no breakfast. Her lunch consisted of salad without dressing and her dinner of plain steamed vegetables and a thin slice of dry wholewheat toast. She ate nothing else at all. No yoghurt, no soya products, no beans, lentils or nuts – the protein-rich foods which her body so badly needed.

After some persuading, because Lesley was afraid to eat more calories, I put her on the Waterfall Diet. Within two weeks, she had lost 4 lb, in spite of eating more food than before. Her weight slowly continued towards normal on the diet and with its help she was able to eat enough protein while remaining vegan.

Protein deficiency questionnaire

- Do you regularly avoid eating meat, dairy products or eggs?
- Do you often miss proper meals and snack instead on chocolate, crisps or chips (French fries)?
- Do you often eat meals consisting of just salad vegetables or fruit and vegetables?
- If you are a vegan, do you eat dishes combining rice with soya, beans, lentils or nuts less than once a day?
- Have you eaten fewer than 1,000 calories a day for more than a few months?

If you answer 'yes' to two or more of these questions, there is a possibility that your water retention may be partly due to protein deficiency.

How does a lack of protein cause water retention?

After a protein-rich meal, your liver uses amino acids to make a type of protein called albumin, which it sends to your blood circulation. Like a magnet, albumin attracts water from your tissues into your blood and prevents water from leaking out of your blood into your tissues. So, if not enough albumin is present, fluid will accumulate in your tissues.

A lack of protein can make you gain weight in another way, too. Protein is needed to make hormones, such as the thyroid hormone which helps to keep your metabolism ticking over. One of the first signs of thyroid hormone deficiency can be weight gain as your metabolism slows down.

Other effects of protein deficiency

The most severe form of protein deficiency (mainly seen in the developing world) is known as kwashiorkor. It is very serious in children, since it retards their growth.

Other protein deficiency effects include impaired digestion, muscle wasting and anaemia. Protein is needed to make digestive enzymes, without which your body cannot absorb the food you consume. If you don't eat enough protein for your body to make its vital hormones and enzymes, your body will start to break down its own muscle tissue. This causes wasting of the arms and legs, while the tummy may look large if it is swollen with water retention.

Balance is essential

Despite the emphasis on protein in this chapter, it is not a good idea to eat only protein in an effort to lose weight more quickly. Too much protein dehydrates you and damages your kidneys. Since you need well-functioning kidneys in order to rid yourself of any fluid you are retaining, you should do everything you can to keep them happy and healthy (*for more on this, see the following chapter*). Always balance protein with vegetables, grains and other dietary essentials.

Case report: Susan ate more protein and lost more pounds

A protein deficiency can be caused by eating a very low-calorie diet, even if it seems to contain enough protein. Forty-eight-year-old Susan weighed 11 stone (154 lb) and for five years had been trying to lose weight through a punishing regime. She got up at six every morning to run for half an hour before leaving for work. She went without breakfast and without lunch. In the evening, she told me, she usually ate a salad with a tinned sardine and a teaspoon of sunflower seeds. She never ate sugar, butter or other fats or oils, and drank only tea with milk.

Susan also had a number of troubling symptoms, including severely flaking fingernails, reduced sex drive and increasing tiredness. She was simply not eating enough food to keep her metabolism and hormones working properly. Grown women need about 2 oz (55 g) of protein a day, which was not being supplied by her single sardine.

Susan was another person terrified of eating more calories. The advice I gave conflicted with that of every other slimming expert she had consulted. It was fortunate that when I put her on the Waterfall Diet and made her promise to eat three meals a day, she lost several pounds almost immediately.

Working with Susan was very rewarding. After two months, she was eating twice as much, weighing 7 lb less and feeling much more energetic. Her husband was also extremely pleased: she confessed that her sex drive had returned – something she had never expected. I discharged her from my care when she was ready to start Phase III of the diet and we both fully expected her weight loss to continue.

Some facts about protein

What is protein?
Protein is the material from which most of your body is made – muscle, hormones, enzymes, skin, hair, organs and the fabric of your bones to which calcium clings are all different types of protein. When you eat protein it is digested into its smallest units, amino acids, which are then absorbed into your bloodstream and help you grow (if you are a child) or repair tissue and make hormones, enzymes and other important substances. If necessary, amino acids can also be converted into energy.

Which foods are rich in protein?
High-protein foods include meat, fish, eggs, milk, yoghurt, cheese, soya products, pulses or legumes (lentils and beans) and nuts.

Rice and other grains are also useful sources of amino acids, but the protein of plants is often called 'incomplete' because it is low in some of the essential amino acids. For example, grains and seeds are low in lysine, whilst pulses and soya products are low in methionine.

Vegetarians and vegans

By eating a variety of plant proteins, we can still get all the amino acids we need without having to resort to eating animal products like meat and cheese. For example, the lysine lacking in rice can be made up for by eating rice with lentils or with other legumes or pulses, since these are rich in lysine. According to the American Dietetic Association, it is probably not necessary to eat them at the same meal. Rice is an ideal accompaniment to beans and lentils, since unlike most other plant foods it is rich in the essential amino acid methionine.

As you can see, you need not develop a protein deficiency if you are vegetarian or vegan. In fact it is generally considered that vegetarians are healthier than the rest of the population.

Protein deficiency and fasting

Protein deficiency also results from simply not eating, as in the case of starvation, anorexia nervosa or long-term fasting for religious or therapeutic purposes. Your body will then begin to break down its own muscle tissue to get the amino acids it needs, and will also slow down its metabolism to minimise its protein needs and muscle breakdown. Some researchers report that the metabolism can slow down by as much as 45 per cent. It is not known how long the body takes to return to a normal rate of metabolism or whether it ever does so completely.

Severe dieting can also slow down your metabolism. If carried out repeatedly, 'yo-yo' dieting can have a cumulative effect on your ability to use calories, so that eventually you could start to gain weight on a calorie intake that never caused you problems before.

How much protein do we need?

Children need more protein than adults. But after the age of nineteen your protein need stops increasing and remains about 2 oz (55 g) a day for a medium-sized man and 1½ oz (45 g) a day for a medium-sized woman.

Protein content of some popular high-protein foods

Food	Protein content
1 chicken leg without skin	26 g
Batter-fried cod portion 4 oz (115 g)	20 g
1 large egg, raw or boiled	6 g
Cheddar cheese 1 oz (28 g)	7 g
Oil-roasted, salted peanuts 3½ oz (100 g)	26 g
Rice, cooked 3½ oz (100 g)	3 g
Tofu 3½ oz (100 g)	8 g
Unsalted, dry, roasted cashew nuts 3½ oz (100 g)	15 g
Yoghurt, plain low-fat 3½ oz (100 g)	7 g

CHAPTER 4

Your personal waterfall: Making your kidneys work for you

Your kidneys are the most important organ for controlling your fluid balance. If you had no kidneys, all the fluid you drink would accumulate in your blood and around your body's cells and all the waste products normally excreted by your kidneys would stay inside you and poison you. You would become very ill and soon die.

Kidney stress over many years can reduce the kidneys' ability to siphon excess fluid out of your body. As we shall see, the major causes of kidney stress include eating too much salt, sugar, protein or fat, and deficiencies of vitamin B_6 and the minerals magnesium and selenium. Mercury (as found in tooth fillings) and other toxic substances can also harm your kidneys.

This chapter looks at what your kidneys need from you to help them remain as stress-free as possible. The Waterfall Diet is ideal for this.

Case report: Sally loved salt

Sally was not overweight, but had been diagnosed with an illness known as psoriatic arthritis. This is a combination of painful joints (in Sally's case mainly her fingers) and the skin disease known as psoriasis. Since painful joints are often caused by water retention, I put her on the Waterfall Diet to see what would happen.

I was really expecting Sally's condition to improve, but two weeks later her joint pains were as bad as ever. Then I discovered that she had been unwittingly cheating. While the diet forbade salt, I had forgotten to tell her that she must not eat smoked fish and kippers – foods with a high salt content. Sally had been eating these every day, complaining that otherwise her meals were too bland. It turned out that she loved salt and had always sprinkled her food liberally with it even when it was already salted. Unsalted food would get a double helping.

Sally spent a very unhappy few days eating food which she did not much enjoy at all, but she soon gained the tremendous benefit of pain-free fingers. Such early relief gave her the incentive to persevere. She also lost 3 lb in weight very quickly, which, as her calorie consumption was not much less than usual, could only be explained by the reduction in her salt intake. As we shall see, salt plays a key role in your fluid balance because it dictates how your kidneys behave. The salt in Sally's diet was interfering with her kidneys, and the resulting water retention was making her fingers hurt.

Answer the following questionnaire to see if your water retention could be related to kidney stress.

Kidney health questionnaire

- Do your ankles regularly swell, especially after you have drunk a lot of liquid?
- Do you put two or more spoonfuls of sugar in your tea or coffee?

- Do you consume cola, lemonade, sugared commercial 'fruit drinks', milk shakes or other sugary drinks every day?
- Do you eat sweets, chocolate, ice-cream or other sugary items several times every day?
- Do you normally consume bread, pastry, cakes, biscuits and pasta made from white flour?
- Do you regularly eat more than 12 ounces a day of high-protein foods such as meat, fish, poultry or cheese?
- Do you eat a lot of fried or greasy food or burgers?
- Do you usually eat highly salted food or add a lot of salt to your food?
- Do you usually eat fresh vegetables or salad vegetables less than once a day?
- Are you vegetarian or vegan?
- Do you have a lot of silver (amalgam) tooth fillings?
- Do you have bowel motions less than once a day?
- Have you ever been diagnosed with a kidney problem?

If you have answered 'yes' to the first question, there is a possibility that your water retention may be partially due to kidney stress. If you have answered 'yes' to any of the other questions, this may help you to pinpoint what might be causing the stress to your kidneys.

The kidneys' tasks

- Maintaining water balance.
- Excreting toxins and waste products.
- Regulating the levels of chemical substances such as sodium, potassium and chloride.
- Regulating blood pressure.
- Adjusting the body's acid–alkaline balance by selecting which ions to retain and which to excrete.

How your kidneys work

All the blood in your body passes through your kidneys about twenty times an hour. Your kidneys' job is to filter your blood, removing excess fluid and the waste substances dissolved in it and sending it to your bladder, where it is known as urine. Normally the more fluid you drink, the more urine your kidneys will produce. If your fluid intake drops, your kidneys will produce less urine.

Your kidneys lie just above your waist on either side of your spine and under the muscles of your back. They are delicate and therefore protected by a cushion of fat. Each kidney consists of about 1.25 million nephrons, tiny units which comprise a filtering apparatus (glomerulus) and a long tube or tubule (*see diagram on p.34*). The glomerulus is actually a dense clump of blood capillaries with a funnel-like structure around it. Fluid and dissolved substances drip out of the porous walls of these capillaries and are collected by the funnel. The fluid drains down through the neck of the funnel into the tubule, which eventually links up with other tubules, all carrying the fluid (now known as urine) towards a larger duct which takes it to the bladder.

Under normal circumstances, the glomeruli filter about 48 gallons (180 litres) of fluid from your blood every day, but of course you do not excrete that much urine. The reason is that certain hormones tell your kidneys how much fluid must be reabsorbed by the tubules and sent back to the blood before your urine reaches the main collecting ducts. If it were not for these hormones, all the fluid in your body would be urinated away within thirty minutes!

The hormones that control your kidneys

The balance of water in your blood is governed by natural hormones that control how much water your kidneys excrete and therefore how much urine you produce.

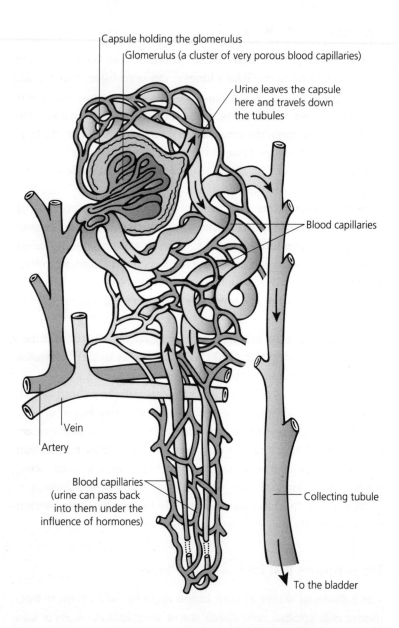

Capsule holding the glomerulus

Glomerulus (a cluster of very porous blood capillaries)

Urine leaves the capsule here and travels down the tubules

Blood capillaries

Vein

Artery

Blood capillaries (urine can pass back into them under the influence of hormones)

Collecting tubule

To the bladder

The nephron: your kidney consists of more than a million of these

Anti-diuretic hormone (ADH)

ADH is secreted by the hypothalamus gland and is stored in your pituitary gland. Both of these glands are located in your head. ADH's job is to reduce urine production when your blood is starting to get dehydrated. Its name should help you to remember what effect it has: 'diuretic' means encouraging the excretion of urine. So 'anti-diuretic' means having the opposite effect.

How it works

When ADH levels are low in your blood, the kidney tubules collect fluid from your blood and send most of it to your bladder. But when ADH is present it makes the tubules porous so they allow some water to filter back into your blood instead of going to your bladder.

Aldosterone

This hormone is made by the adrenal glands, situated on top of your kidneys. Like ADH, it is released in order to reduce urine production when your blood is beginning to get dehydrated.

How it works

Aldosterone makes the kidney tubules hold on to some of the sodium in the fluid passing through them and draw this sodium back into your blood circulation. Sodium always pulls water along with it, so provided that ADH has prepared your tubules by making them porous, water will leave the tubules to return to your blood before it reaches your bladder.

The rule that water follows sodium applies in more ways than one. Consuming too much sodium, in the form of table salt, or as additives (such as monosodium glutamate) in soft drinks and processed foods, forces your body to crave more and more fluid. Just as in Sally's case, your body will retain this fluid until it has the chance to excrete the excess sodium.

The use of diuretics

Doctors treat water retention by prescribing drugs which will stop the kidney tubules from reabsorbing sodium. If less sodium is reabsorbed then less water will be reabsorbed, and so more water will be excreted. These drugs, known as diuretics, have a number of side-effects. In preventing sodium reabsorption, many of them will also prevent the reabsorption of other essential minerals such as potassium and magnesium. Deficiencies of these important nutrients can then develop. Physical side-effects include dry mouth and rashes, and the drugs can also lead to kidney damage and to a worsening of any pre-existing diabetes or gout.

Drastically reducing your salt intake can help you to avoid or reduce diuretic drugs – with your doctor's permission, of course. If you are already taking these drugs, whether or not you can safely come off them depends on why your doctor has prescribed them. If your water retention is due to a heart problem, for instance, you will probably need to stay on them.

Atrial natriuretic hormone (ANH) and dopamine

There are two more important hormones involved in kidney function. One, relatively newly discovered, is known as atrial natriuretic hormone (ANH) and is secreted by the heart. The other hormone, dopamine, has only recently been discovered to have an effect on water balance.

Both ANH and dopamine have the opposite effect to aldosterone. They encourage water excretion by preventing you from reabsorbing sodium.

Levels of all these natural hormones are constantly being adjusted in your body in order to help ensure that the amount of water in your blood remains at an ideal level.

Water retention and minerals

As you can see, sodium plays a vital role in how your body fluid behaves. Your kidneys filter sodium out of your blood and then return sodium to your blood in the exact amount that your body needs. When sodium levels rise, as when you eat salted foods, thirst makes you drink so that the sodium in your blood will not be too concentrated. Then your kidneys excrete the extra water and the extra sodium together.

Why do your kidneys exert such careful control over sodium?

The answer is in the job which sodium and other minerals have to do. Two-thirds of your body's fluid has to reside inside your cells and one-third outside. If this balance is disrupted, your cells could burst by absorbing too much water. Alternatively, they would collapse if they did not get enough water. Levels of sodium and other minerals control this water balance. Water is attracted to minerals, so if the mineral concentrations inside and outside your cells are correct, the proportions of water should also be correct.

Minerals attract water by means of tiny electrical charges formed when they dissolve in water. These electrical charges also decide whether the minerals end up inside or outside your cells. When minerals are dissolved in water they separate into positively charged sodium particles (ions) and negatively charged chloride particles. This water can then conduct electricity. Nerve cells are especially dependent on electrical charges to carry messages to your brain, spinal cord and muscles. Those minerals which play an important role due to their ability to carry electrical charges are known as electrolytes.

Your diet and your kidneys

We have all heard about the foods we should or should not eat to help prevent clogged arteries which could lead to a heart attack, but rarely do we hear any dietary advice for the benefit of our kidneys. Yet a lot of research has been done into the effects of various foods on the health of our kidneys. Since your kidneys play such a vital role in helping you to excrete excess fluid, you could benefit from paying attention to these research findings if you think you may be suffering from water retention.

Salt and sugar

As we have already seen, consuming too much salt is a direct cause of water retention. Salt is hidden in many convenience foods and is even found in bread. Manufacturers are reducing the amount of salt they add to food, but on the whole most experts agree that we still eat too much salt. (*You can find more information about salt and its health effects on pp.45–6.*)

A possibly even more damaging dietary habit, in terms of kidney health, is the number of sugary foods and drinks we consume as a nation. Most of us eat about 2 lb (almost a kilogram) of sugar a week (usually without realising it) in the form of:

  sweets and chocolate
  sweetened tea and coffee
  soft drinks
  breakfast cereals
  jam, marmalade, honey, syrup
  cakes
  biscuits
  ice cream

Not only can sugar encourage the kidneys to retain sodium (which could make you retain fluid), but it also has a directly damaging effect on your kidneys and could in time lead to enlarged kidneys and kidney stones.

Sugar and kidney damage

Dr N. J. Blacklock from the University Hospital of South Manchester in England is one of the world's top experts on diet and kidney function. In a 1986 research study he gave 250 grams (about 9 oz) of sugar a day to a group of volunteers and then measured levels of a chemical known as NAG, which is produced by the body when damage has occurred to the kidney tubules. In every case NAG levels were higher after the sugar was consumed.

Over the years, the damage caused by sugar can build up, making your kidneys less efficient and even enlarging them as they try to compensate for the damage. Once kidney damage becomes extensive, whatever its cause, scar tissue can replace your nephrons – that is, your normal kidney tissue.

While the amount of sugar used in Dr Blacklock's study seems like a lot, remember that the average sugar consumption in the UK is just over 4 oz (115 g) a day. So while a lot of people are consuming less than this, an equally large number are consuming more. When I was a child, I could easily get through 8 oz (227 g) of sweets in a day – that is 8 oz of pure sugar! I dread to think what effect this kind of diet is having on some young people's kidneys.

Sugar and kidney stones

Dr N. J. Blacklock is also concerned about the effects of sugar on kidney stone formation. About one-third of the population produces very high levels of the hormone insulin when they consume sugar, he says, and this excess of insulin makes kidneys excrete more calcium. This excess calcium can then form hard tiny plugs or 'stones' in the kidney tubules (*see diagram on p.40*). If the stones grow they can get 'stuck' and cause great pain, especially when they shift with the flow of fluid. The treatment of choice for kidney stones is to help them to pass along the tubules and into the bladder. If this does not work, surgery or ultrasound treatment may be required.

High insulin levels caused by consuming sugary foods and drinks can also make the kidneys retain sodium. As we have

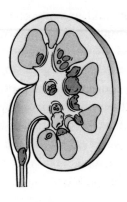

Kidney stones

already seen, sodium retention leads to water retention. Diabetics who have to use insulin injections are also prone to water retention for the same reason.

The importance of vitamin B_6 and magnesium

Kidney stones are more likely to form if you have a deficiency of vitamin B_6 and of the mineral magnesium. At least three medical journals, *Urology Research*, the prestigious French journal *Presse Médicale*, and *International Urology and Nephrology*, have published reports that people with a higher intake of these two nutrients have a much reduced risk of developing kidney stones, so it really is worth taking good nutrition seriously. Only if your kidneys are healthy can they work as efficiently as possible to filter your blood and get rid of excess water.

To get more vitamin B_6 and magnesium you need to eat wholegrains, nuts, beans and leafy green vegetables. The Waterfall Diet helps you to get more of these foods.

Protein, fat and fibre

In 1982, the *British Journal of Urology* reported a study in which 392 kidney-stone patients were given a diet high in dietary fibre and low in sugar, white flour and animal protein. Their kidneys began to excrete much lower amounts of calcium, oxalate and uric acid – all signs that their kidneys were healthier and less likely to develop kidney stones.

Fibre is especially important, as it helps your kidneys by reducing their workload and by preventing constipation. As you will see in Chapter 6, constipation can raise the amounts of harmful waste products in your blood and create a much heavier workload for your kidneys. Foods rich in dietary fibre include porridge oats, beans, wholemeal bread and brown rice.

Selenium and your kidneys

One very interesting research study was reported in 1990 in the *Journal of Trace Elements and Electrolytes in Health and Disease*. Eleven healthy volunteers at the Laboratory of Clinical Chemistry in Valeggio, Italy, were given selenium supplements at doses of up to 700 micrograms a day (one microgram is a thousandth of a milligram, which in turn is one thousandth of a gram) by Dr Guidi and his team. When the doctors measured how well their kidneys were working, they found that levels of creatinine, a waste substance found in the blood, had dropped by 13 per cent – a very clear indication that the kidneys were working much more efficiently.

Selenium is a trace element which your body requires in tiny amounts: about 75 micrograms a day. Selenium protects against carcinogenic substances, activates your thyroid hormone and helps you to make an antioxidant enzyme that protects against heart disease and viruses. The Italian study seems to be the first to suggest that selenium is also important for kidney function.

Another interesting study was carried out on rats in 1995 at the Swedish Institute for Genetic and Cellular Toxicology, University of Stockholm. After giving the rats a selenium-deficient diet, Dr U. Olsson and colleagues noticed that the rats' normal kidney function became progressively disturbed.

In the UK, the soil is very poor in selenium, so very little is found in crops. Bread used to make up for this when much of the wheat for flour-making was imported from Canada, a country with selenium-rich soil. But European Union regulations mean that the UK must now use mainly EU wheat, and as a result the nation's average selenium consumption has dropped to about 30 micrograms a day – less than half the recommended necessary intake of 75 micrograms, and even below the amount officially classed as inadequate.

Mercury – a kidney toxin

Another beneficial effect which selenium supplementation may have on your kidneys is to reduce your body's levels of the toxic metal mercury. Dr G. N. Schrauzer's research was reported in the German medical journal *Deutsche Zeitschrift für Biologische Zahnmedizin* in 1989. Mercury is found in silver (amalgam) tooth fillings and over the years is known to leak out in minute amounts into your blood. As your kidneys filter the blood, the mercury accumulates in them because it is extremely hard to excrete.

Several medical and dental journals have now reported that the more amalgam fillings are in the mouth, the more mercury can collect in the kidneys. For instance, researchers at the University of Umea in Sweden have found that mercury levels rose continuously after amalgam fillings were placed for the first time in eight healthy individuals. A study reported in the *Swedish Dental Journal* in 1987 found that when the bodies of twelve people were examined at autopsy, those with amalgam fillings had much higher levels of mercury in their kidneys than those without.

Studies carried out on sheep (an animal chosen because it spends much of its time chewing) by Canadian dental researcher Murray Vimy suggest that an average number of amalgam fillings could over a lifetime destroy half your kidney cells. That's not good news. As we've already seen, healthy kidneys are needed for a healthy water balance in your body.

The good news is that selenium helps you to excrete mercury by binding to it. But to be on the safe side, many people are having their silver fillings gradually replaced with white ones or with inlays. Most fillings eventually need replacing anyway. When silver fillings are removed, ask your dentist to use a rubber dam to prevent you from absorbing any mercury during this process. And do not swallow it.

Do remember, all dentists agree that the best way to avoid fillings is to avoid sugary foods.

How to get more selenium

If kidneys work better with more selenium, it would certainly make sense to start taking supplements, since in the UK there seems no other way to increase our selenium intake to a healthy level. Apart from meat and fish, the only other good natural source is Brazil nuts, but you would need to eat between ten and twenty a day to raise your selenium intake from 30 to 75 micrograms. Dr Guidi's Italian patients were presumably also eating a diet deficient in selenium, and this is why the supplements helped them.

The generally preferred forms of selenium supplementation are selenium-rich yeast and L-selenomethionine. Supplements of these products are considered perfectly safe at levels of up to 200 micrograms a day. Another supplement which (very slowly) helps to carry excess mercury out of the body is the amino acid n-acetyl cysteine (NAC), also available as supplements.

Getting the balance right

Don't be surprised if you are starting to feel confused about the 'ideal' diet. As we saw in Chapter 3, too little protein causes water retention. Now we find that too much protein stresses the kidneys. Too little fat is bad for you – and too much fat is also bad for you. How can the average person get it right?

While most of the dietary advice you will need is in Section II, here are a couple of helpful tips to be going on with:

- The bulk of your food should be minimally processed. That is to say, eat brown rice in preference to white, and wholemeal bread instead of white, nine times out of ten. Apart from other nutrients, these foods are rich in vitamin B_6, magnesium and dietary fibre – all good for your kidneys.
- Whenever possible, prepare your food from scratch instead of buying convenience foods. That way you know how much fat and sugar it contains and you can control your intake of these items more easily.

Medical research is showing again and again that a diet based on the principles of the Waterfall Diet will protect your kidneys from the illnesses and malfunctions that so often come with age and lead to water retention.

And don't worry if you have bad habits now; it is never too late to reap the benefits of changing them.

Some facts about salt

Only 10 per cent of the salt in our diet comes from the natural salt in foods. The rest comes from adding salt to food. Salt is used both as a condiment in cookery and as a food additive and pre-servative. Foods high in salt include bacon, ham, salami, sausages, pork pies and other preserved meats, canned fish, smoked fish, soy sauce, yeast extract, many cheeses, salted butter, salted peanuts and other packet snacks, packet and canned soups and sauces, bread, stock cubes and ready-cooked meals for reheating. The reg-ular consumption of these foods, plus the salt added to your food, can easily lead to an intake of 12–17 grams a day. But the World Health Organization recommends no more than 5 grams. Recent

government guidelines in the UK have encouraged the food industry to reduce salt in many products, but the Food Standards
Agency says our average salt consumption is still too high.

Salt and your health
A high salt intake has been linked with high blood pressure and
strokes. This is because the sodium in salt encourages water retention, and too much water in your arteries raises the pressure
inside them. But not all individuals with high blood pressure
respond to a low-salt diet – some are thought to be more salt-sen-
sitive than others.

Recent research shows that a high salt intake encourages
osteoporosis (brittle bone disease). Salt also seems to increase
the lungs' sensitivity to histamine, and studies have shown that
asthma is worsened by a high salt intake.

As described by Dr Nadya Coates in her book *A Matter of Life*
(Optima, 1990), sodium chloride, in contact with water, breaks
down in your body to hydrochloric acid and caustic soda. The
hydrochloric acid is removed from your blood and used in your
digestion processes. The sodium hydroxide remains as an irritant
to your cells and has to be neutralised with lactic acid. Severe
sodium hydroxide irritation may be experienced as a burning sensation in the affected parts of the body, even though these parts
may feel cold to the touch. Some authorities believe that the
resultant damage to cells could act as a trigger for cancer.

It's easy to cut down
You can reduce your salt intake by avoiding high-salt foods, by
exercising caution with all foods not prepared at home (especially
if they taste salty) and by using low-sodium salt or salt substitute
(*usually potassium chloride, see p.192*) in cooking and at the
table.

The zinc link

Children who are faddy eaters and eat only sweet or highly salted foods may have had their sense of taste damaged by a zinc deficiency. It is quite hard to get substantial amounts of zinc from your diet unless you eat mostly wholegrain foods, lentils, beans, nuts, meat and fish. So zinc deficiency is becoming increasingly common. To zinc-deficient people, most foods taste too bland unless plenty of salt or other flavouring is added. Once the zinc deficiency has been corrected, your child may begin to enjoy a wider range of foods.

Organic sodium may be good for you

Salt (in chemical terms, sodium chloride) is not the only source of sodium in your diet. Most natural foods contain only a small sodium content, but it is probably beneficial. The best sources are fresh fish, meat, eggs, celery, beetroot, carrots, radishes, spinach and watercress. Sodium occurring in such foods is normally found incorporated in plant or animal cells and is therefore in organic form and may be handled differently by the human body when consumed.

We should point out that 'organic' is not used here in the usual sense of food grown without pesticides and fertilisers. An organic mineral is found in living tissues as opposed to the minerals found in rocks, for example.

The organic sodium found in vegetables such as celery may help to keep inorganic sodium (from salt) dissolved, thus helping your body to eliminate it. In Section II of this book you will see that celery and celery juice are special Waterfall Diet foods and you will be encouraged to consume them as often as possible.

CHAPTER 5

The medicines that can make you fat: What is your doctor prescribing?

Water retention can be a side-effect of a surprisingly large number of both necessary and unnecessary prescription medicines, particularly female hormonal treatments, painkillers, steroids and blood pressure medications.

> Under the law, proof is not required that a medicine be safe, only that its benefits should outweigh its side-effects.

Case report: Jean's prescription piled on the pounds

Jean consulted me as a last resort. 'My doctor says I've got to lose weight for my blood pressure,' she said, 'otherwise my heart could get damaged. He sent me to the dietician, who gave me a 1000-calorie-a-day diet, but I was already eating less than that, so I'm gaining weight on it. What can I do? He won't believe me when I tell him how little I'm eating.'

Poor Jean was very distressed. One of the first things I noticed was her swollen ankles, so I immediately suspected that she was retaining fluid. 'How long have they been swollen?' I asked. Jean replied that she had first become aware of them soon after beginning to take the beta blocker drugs her doctor had given her for her blood pressure. It turned out that the weight gain had also started around this time. I asked Jean some more questions designed to find out if she was an allergic type or possibly deficient in protein, but the drugs remained the only clue to her problem.

Medical reference books confirmed that beta blockers could indeed cause water retention, but Jean's doctor had not put two and two together. Although Jean seemed very nervous of questioning his advice, she promised to get up the courage to return, show him her swollen ankles and discuss the possibility that her weight gain might be due to the medication.

Answer the following questionnaire to see if prescription medicines could be causing your water retention.

Medicines questionnaire

- Are you taking any of the medicines described in the table overleaf?
- Did the start of your water retention/weight gain seem to coincide with beginning to take this medicine?
- Has your water retention/weight gain worsened since you started to take this medicine?
- Have you ever taken any of the medicines described as causing possible kidney damage?
- Has your water retention/weight gain only become noticeable since the time when you took this drug?

Drugs which can promote water retention

Drug type (generic name)	Some common brand names	Used mainly for	Effects on fluid balance	Possible alternatives
ACE Inhibitors: e.g. Captopril	Acepril, Capoten	High blood pressure and congestive heart failure	Toxic to kidneys. May also cause swellings due to allergic water retention	Nutritional therapy Herbal therapy
Beta blockers: e.g. Metoprolol Pindolol Propranolol	Betaloc, Lopressor Visken Inderal	High blood pressure, angina, anxiety	May reduce the heart's ability to pump the blood through the kidneys, thus encouraging water retention	Nutritional therapy Herbal therapy Relaxation techniques
Calcium channel blockers: e.g. Nifedipine	Adalat Adipine Cardilate MR Coracten Unipine XL	Angina, high blood pressure, Raynaud's disease	May reduce the heart's ability to pump the blood through the kidneys, thus encouraging water retention	Nutritional therapy Herbal therapy Homoeopathy
Central Alpha Stimulant: Clonidine Methyldopa	Catapres, Dixarit, Aldomet	High blood pressure, migraine, menopausal hot flushes	Can cause sodium retention and consequent water retention	Nutritional therapy Herbal therapy Homoeopathy Traditional Chinese medicine
Vasodilators: e.g. Diazoxide Hydralazine Minoxidil	Eudemine Apresoline Loniten, Regaine	High blood pressure. Regaine is sometimes used to treat male baldness	May reduce the heart's ability to pump the blood through the kidneys, thus encouraging water retention	Nutritional therapy Herbal therapy

Table continued ▶

Drugs which can promote water retention

Drug type (generic name)	Some common brand names	Used mainly for	Effects on fluid balance	Possible alternatives
Reserpine	No longer used in the UK but still used in some countries	High blood pressure	Can cause sodium retention and consequent water retention	Nutritional therapy Herbal therapy
Loop diuretics: e.g. Bumetanide Frusemide	Burinex Lasix	Water retention	Capable of causing kidney damage. All diuretics can worsen high-protein type water retention	While there are several herbal diuretics, these will not solve the underlying problem causing the fluid retention. See Chapter 9 for dealing with the causes
Thiazide diuretics	Hygroton Saluric	Water retention	Capable of causing kidney damage. All diuretics can worsen high-protein type water retention	While there are several herbal diuretics, these will not solve the underlying problem causing the fluid retention. See Chapter 9 for dealing with the causes
Potassium-sparing diuretics	Dytac Amilamont Amilospare Berkamil	Water retention	All diuretics can worsen high-protein water retention	While there are several herbal diuretics, these will not solve the underlying problem causing the fluid retention. See Chapter 9 for dealing with the causes

Drugs which can promote water retention

Drug type (generic name)	Some common brand names	Used mainly for	Effects on fluid balance	Possible alternatives
NSAIDS: e.g. Aceclophenac Acemetacin Aspirin-type painkillers Azapropazone Diclofenac sodium Diflunisal Etodolac Fenbufen Fenoprofen Flurbiprofen Ibuprofen Indomethacin Ketoprofen Ketorolac Mefenamic acid Meloxicam Nabumetone Naproxen Phenylbutazone Piroxicam Sulindac Tenoxicam Tiapofenic acid Tolmetin	Preservex Emflex Anadin, Nuseals Rheumox Voltarol, Diclomax Dolobid Lodine Lederfen Fenopron Froben, Ocufen Brufen, Nurofen, Cuprofen Indocid, Flexin Ketofen, Oruvail, Orudis Acular, Toradol Ponstan, Meflam Mobic Reliflex Naprosyn, Synflex, Naprotec Butacote Feldene Clinoril Mobiflex Surgam Tolectin	Pain and inflammation	Prevent production of prostaglandins involved in kidney function	Nutritional therapy Herbal therapy Acupuncture Homoeopathy
Corticosteroid Drugs: e.g. Beclomethasone Betamethasone Dexamethasone Fludrocortisone Flunisolide Prednisone } Prednisolone } Triamcinolone	Becotide, Becloforte Betnesol Decadron, Maxidex Florinef Syntaris Deltacortril, Precortisyl Forte Adcortyl, Kenalog, Nasocort	Pain and inflammation, asthma	Can cause sodium retention and consequent water retention	Nutritional therapy Herbal therapy Acupuncture Homoeopathy

Table continued ▶

Drugs which can promote water retention

Drug type (generic name)	Some common brand names	Used mainly for	Effects on fluid balance	Possible alternatives
Amphotericin	Fungilin, Ambisone, Fungizone	Anti-fungal	Toxic to the kidneys	Nutritional therapy
Oestrogen	Premarin, Premique, Prempak	Contraceptive pill and HRT	Causes sodium retention and consequent water retention	There are many alternative methods of contraception
Progestogen	Duphaston, Provera, Primolut, Cyclogest	Contraceptive pill and HRT	Causes sodium retention and consequent water retention	Nutritional therapy, herbal therapy, traditional Chinese medicine and homoeopathy can all help against menopausal problems
Danazol	Danot	Endometriosis	Reasons for water retention are unclear	Nutritional therapy Herbal therapy Traditional Chinese medicine Homoeopathy
Phenothiazines	Largactil, Stelazine	Mental illness	May reduce the heart's ability to pump the blood through the kidneys, thus encouraging water retention	Nutritional therapy is an effective treatment in those many cases of mental illness caused by abnormally high nutritional needs which have gone unfulfilled

Drugs which can promote water retention

Drug type (generic name)	Some common brand names	Used mainly for	Effects on fluid balance	Possible alternatives
Tricyclic anti-depressants: e.g. Amitryptiline Clomipramine Desipramine Imipramine Nortriptyline	Tryptizol, Tryptafen, Lentizol Anafranil Pertofran Tofranil Allegron, Motipress, Motival	Mental illness	Water retention may occur as an allergic reaction	Nutritional therapy
Insulin	Any brand, and also high levels of natural insulin	Diabetes	Can cause sodium retention and consequent water retention	Do not attempt to stop insulin treatment. Nutritional therapy can help but should be used under the supervision of a doctor
Metoclopramide	Maxolon, Paramax, Gastrobid	Nausea, vomiting, migraine	Causes a rise in aldosterone (sodium-retention hormone). May also cause swellings due to allergic water retention	Alternatives depend on treating the causes of these problems
Cephalosporin antibiotics: e.g. Cephaclor	Distaclor	Bacterial infections	Water retention may occur as an allergic reaction	Vitamin C megadoses, raw garlic, herbal anti-bacterials. Use under medical supervision

Table continued ▶

Drugs which can promote water retention

Drug type (generic name)	Some common brand names	Used mainly for	Effects on fluid balance	Possible alternatives
Co-trimoxazole antibiotics	Septrin	Bacterial infections	Capable of causing kidney damage	Vitamin C megadoses, raw garlic, herbal anti-bacterials. Use under medical supervision
Aciclovir anti-virals	Zovirax	Viral infections	Capable of causing kidney damage	Vitamin C megadoses. Uña de gato (cat's claw) herb. Possibly olive leaf extract, though research on humans is lacking

Sources of drug toxicity information: online search of drug databases, American Society of Health drug information, British National Formulary.

The table contains brand names as well as generic drug names and is intended for at-a-glance reference. The descriptions in the text on the following pages contain only generic names (so you may not find your particular medication named here) but offer fuller details.

If you believe that a drug may be causing your water retention, it is very important that you do not come off it without discussing the problem with your doctor.

Drugs used to reduce high blood pressure

As blood is pumped through the arteries, the pressure it exerts against your artery walls is known as your blood pressure. It can be raised above normal by hormonal imbalances, by narrowing of your arteries (which forces your heart to pump harder), by water retention and by excessive stickiness (viscosity) of your blood. High blood pressure must be treated. Doctors normally use drugs which:

- act as diuretics, or
- help to keep the arteries as wide (dilated) as possible, or
- prevent your hormones from quickening your heartbeat.

Captopril

This is a type of drug known as an ACE inhibitor. It is used to treat high blood pressure and congestive heart failure – a condition in which the heart's pumping ability begins to fail. It works by blocking the chain of reactions which produce the hormone aldosterone. As explained in Chapter 4, aldosterone stimulates your kidneys to retain some of the sodium in the fluid passing through them. The sodium is then drawn back into your blood along with water, which reduces urination. By blocking aldosterone, ACE inhibitor drugs make you urinate more, thus reducing the amount of fluid in your blood. This gives your heart less work to do and lowers your blood pressure.

Between 4 and 12 per cent of patients who are prescribed this drug find its side-effects too severe to remain on it. It can cause swellings (localised water retention) and can be quite toxic to the kidneys; doctors are instructed to monitor their patients' kidney function while they are on it.

Pindolol, propranolol and metoprolol

These drugs are known as beta blockers. They are used to treat high blood pressure, angina, anxiety and migraine. They work by preventing the body from responding to stress in its usual way. When stressful emotions (anger, fear, excitement, tension, anxiety and so on) are felt, hormones such as adrenaline (epinephrine in the USA) are released by the body and stimulate the heart to beat faster and harder. Beta blockers reduce this stimulation, slowing down the heart and reducing its pumping force, which helps to keep the blood pressure down. In angina sufferers it helps to prevent pain and in anxiety sufferers it reduces the physical symptoms of anxiety.

Many of the side-effects of beta blockers are related to the slowing down of the heart: coldness and circulatory problems, depression, impotence and memory loss. Between 6 and 16 per cent of people on pindolol suffer from water retention in hands, feet and ankles.

Nifedipine

This is a so-called calcium channel blocker drug, used to treat high blood pressure, angina and the 'cold fingers syndrome' known as Raynaud's disease. The drug decreases the contraction of arteries and veins by blocking the entry of calcium into cells. This keeps these vessels dilated, which reduces the blood pressure and improves the blood flow. Nifedipine is often prescribed together with beta blockers to counteract some of the circulation problems which these drugs produce.

Drug toxicity researchers are worried at the lack of data on the potential adverse effects of calcium channel blocker drugs. The main side-effect, suffered by 10–30 per cent of patients taking nifedipine on a long-term basis, is water retention, especially in the ankles. Also, 25 per cent of patients develop dizziness, light-headedness, flushing or heat sensation and headaches.

Methyldopa and clonidine

These are another type of drug which reduces blood pressure by dilating the arteries. Acting mainly on blood pressure-controlling sites in the brain, they prevent arteries from contracting in response to nerve stimulation. Clonidine is also used to treat menopausal hot flushes and to prevent migraine. Not used much nowadays, both drugs can cause sodium retention which leads to water retention.

Diazoxide, hydralazine and minoxidil

Patients with high blood pressure which does not respond to a combination of beta blocker and diuretic drugs may be given one of these drugs, which act directly on the muscles of the arteries, helping to dilate them. One of their most common side-effects is sodium retention, leading to fluid retention and weight gain.

Minoxidil is also used as a scalp application to treat male-pattern baldness.

Reserpine

Derived from the roots of an Indian climbing shrub known as rawolfia, this drug lowers the blood pressure and slows the heart. It has a sedative effect and was formerly used to treat mental illness. Reserpine can also cause sodium retention and consequent water retention. It is no longer prescribed in the UK but may still be used in some other countries

Drugs used to promote urination (diuretics)

Water retention is one of the factors which promotes high blood pressure. The more fluid the heart has to try to pump around the body, the harder it has to pump and so the greater the pressure exerted on the artery walls. To help reduce this pressure doctors will often prescribe a diuretic drug to prevent the kidney tubules from reabsorbing sodium and water. More water will then be excreted as urine. As we have already seen, many blood pressure-reducing medications also promote water retention, so it is common practice for a doctor to administer a beta blocker and a diuretic together.

Diuretic drugs are also used to treat water retention caused by kidney or liver disease and congestive heart failure. As less blood is pumped through the kidneys, the body starts to retain more and more fluid. If these fluid levels rise too high there is a risk of the body becoming starved of oxygen, so it is essential to reduce them. Doctors do this by administering diuretic drugs.

There are three types of diuretic drugs: loop diuretics, thiazides and potassium-sparing diuretics.

Loop diuretics: bumetanide and frusemide

These drugs are known as loop diuretics because they inhibit sodium reabsorption in a particular section of the kidney tubule known as the loop of Henle. They are very powerful and are known to inhibit the body's reabsorption of potassium, magnesium and calcium, which could cause deficiencies of these important substances.

Although this is not among the most frequent side-effects of bumetanide and frusemide, both drugs are capable of causing kidney damage. Like all diuretics, they could worsen Type II water retention (*see p.98–9*).

Thiazide diuretics

Thiazides comprise the largest group of diuretic drugs and are moderate in potency. Like the loop diuretics, they deplete the body of sodium, magnesium and potassium, and may raise uric acid levels in the blood. They can cause kidney damage and worsen Type II water retention.

Potassium-sparing diuretics: spironolactone, triamterine and amiloride

This group is so called because the drugs it comprises are thought not to result in such large potassium losses from the body as the other types of diuretics. However, they too can worsen Type II water retention.

Painkillers

Two types of drugs are used to treat pain and inflammation, and are prescribed on a long-term basis in conditions such as rheumatoid arthritis. The first type are known as non-steroidal because they are not based on imitations of the body's own steroid hormones; the other type are known as steroidal anti-inflammatory drugs, and are similar to cortisone. It is not widely known that both types of painkillers can promote water retention when used long term.

Non-steroidal anti-inflammatory drugs (NSAIDS)

These drugs have a large number of generic names (*see table on pp.49–54*) and treat pain by blocking the body's production of prostaglandins – hormone-like substances which play a part in causing pain sensations. Prostaglandins are also involved in the kidneys' ability to extract fluid from the blood. Blocking these prostaglandins can result in water retention. Most NSAIDS can also cause some degree of kidney damage when used in high doses regularly on a long-term basis (rather than just for the occasional headache).

Corticosteroid drugs

These steroid drugs, which resemble hormones produced by the body's adrenal glands (situated above the kidneys), are given by mouth to treat rheumatoid arthritis, ulcerative colitis and other inflammatory diseases, and asthma, or may be applied externally as creams or ointments to treat skin inflammations such as eczema. Some corticosteroid drugs such as beclomethasone and fluticasone are also available for asthma patients to inhale. These products include Becotide and Flixotide inhalers. (*Again, see the table on pp.49–54 for generic names.*)

The dangers of steroid drugs are well known, and should not be underestimated. It is especially dangerous to stop taking them suddenly. Regular use of these drugs makes the body stop producing its own corticosteroids and rely on the drugs instead.

Corticosteroids cause water retention by encouraging the body to retain sodium. Other side-effects include shrinkage of the adrenal glands, osteoporosis, susceptibility to infections, thrush, diabetes, mental disturbances such as mood swings, thinning of the skin, acne and the growth of extra body or facial hair.

Anti-fungal drugs

Amphotericin

You may be prescribed amphotericin if you suffer from a fungal or yeast infection such as thrush. It is normally prescribed for six to ten weeks and sometimes longer. Fungal infections can develop in your mouth and throat, intestines or vagina. They are more likely to occur if your immune system is depressed through lack of proper nourishment, from taking immune-suppressing drugs such as corticosteroids, or from a life-threatening condition such as AIDS.

Amphotericin is potentially harmful to the liver and kidneys. This is the reason why it is included here among the list of potential water retention-promoting drugs.

Sex steroids

Oestrogens and progestogens

You may never have heard oestrogens and progestogens (known in the United States as progestins) referred to as steroid drugs before, but this is indeed what they are and how they are classified in medical books. Steroids are hormones with a particular type of chemical structure and these female sex hormones conform to that structure.

Synthetic or semi-synthetic ethinyloestradiol, mestranol and progestogen are normally used in the contraceptive pill rather than the natural hormones oestradiol (the most active form of oestrogen) and progesterone. Although real oestrogen (extracted from urine) can be administered as patches for hormone replacement therapy (HRT), it is not usually given by mouth since it is not well absorbed from the intestines. Progesterone cannot be taken by mouth as it is broken down by the digestion.

The synthetic forms are far more potent than our own natural hormones. Although they are administered in tiny amounts, their effects on the female body are extremely powerful and they are more difficult to break down and excrete.

Synthetic oestrogens and progestogens both encourage sodium retention and therefore water retention. This is a major side-effect of both drugs and can lead to breast tenderness, tummy swelling and a weight gain of several pounds. (*For more on the contraceptive pill and HRT, see pp.64–7.*)

Other drugs

Further drugs which can cause water retention include:

- Tricyclic antidepressants and phenothiazines, used to treat mental illness.
- The antiviral drug aciclovir.
- Danazol, a masculinising drug given for endometriosis.
- Insulin, which is essential for the treatment of insulin-dependent diabetes.
- Metoclopramide, used to treat nausea, vomiting and migraine.
- Some antibiotics, which are occasionally toxic to the kidneys but are more likely to cause water retention by provoking an allergic reaction.

It should be remembered that any drug, like any food, can cause allergic symptoms in sensitive individuals, and that allergy can result in considerable water retention (*see Chapter 2*).

Taking responsibility for your health

In natural medicine, we talk about taking responsibility for your health as the first step in preventing or combating health problems like water retention. Taking responsibility for your health means treating your body with respect and understanding that whether it functions well for you or not often depends on how well you obey natural laws which you cannot change. Natural medicine practitioners try to help people understand the limitations of drug-based medicine and particularly its dangers. Here are a few issues to consider.

Do I really need my drugs?

Only your doctor can answer this question, but not unless you ask. Asking him/her the following questions can help you to make more informed decisions about your treatments:

- 'Is my problem serious enough to need medical treatment right now?'
- 'Will your treatment cure it or just help me to cope with it?'
- 'Is my problem likely to get worse even if I take your treatment?'
- 'What side-effects does your treatment have?'

In case your doctor wishes to shield you from knowing about all the potential side-effects of the recommended medicine (because you might start imagining you develop them!), you should also do your own research to discover the potential side-effects. Your local pharmacist will have a reference book where you can look them up. Other books will be available through your local reference library.

It may be that although you cannot come off your medication right now, you might be able to if you obtain an improvement in your condition by using natural medicine.

Do alternatives work as well as conventional medicine?

That depends on what your health problem is and what you are trying to achieve. If all you want is a painkiller for an occasional headache, conventional medicine provides a cheap, effective and convenient solution. But if you have arthritis which is slowly getting worse, or migraine attacks every week, the treatment is still basically only painkillers. With a few notable exceptions such as antibiotics, most medical treatments do nothing to stem the progress of an illness. They only act as palliatives, helping you to cope with it a little more easily provided that you continue taking the medication every day. As soon as you stop taking it, the palliative effect is lost. This means that most medical treatments are not, in fact, effective in achieving what you want – which is presumably to stop or reverse the illness rather than just control the symptoms.

Natural medicine, on the other hand, is capable of real cures for chronic illnesses. Nutritional therapy can be especially effective, since so much ill health – including most of the health problems named in this chapter – is caused by faulty nutrition and so can be reversed by giving your body what it needs. The principle is the same as when you treat an ailing plant by giving it more minerals or changing it to a lime-rich soil. The cells in your body have much in common with plants.

Because it is so nourishing, following the Waterfall Diet is likely to bring you more benefits than just reducing water retention. You will probably sleep better and have better skin, more energy and fewer headaches. If you are a woman, problems like period pains and PMS can disappear. More serious health problems such as asthma, arthritis and high blood pressure can also improve, although for these you may need a more tailored nutritional treatment, obtainable from a nutritional therapist (*see Useful Addresses on p.276*).

If you decide to try a particular natural therapy, do tell your doctor in case there are any objections. If he/she has any worries, your natural therapist should be able to supply you with information to reassure him/her. Not only are therapies like nutritional therapy very well backed up by science, but consumer surveys (for instance, the 1995 UK Consumers' Association study) carried out on people who have used natural therapies show that the vast majority find them helpful and good value for money. If you or your doctor are interested in nutritional therapy research, see my website (www.health-diets.net). Finally, don't allow yourself to feel intimidated by your doctor or to be afraid of getting a second opinion. There is sure to be a doctor in your area who is interested in natural medicine or even employs natural medical practitioners in his/her practice.

Is bad health really preventable?

Most things become preventable when we understand what causes them and are able to influence those causes. Unfortunately, the majority of doctors are poorly informed about nutritional therapy and natural medicine. It is almost impossible for practitioners of low-technology medicine to compete with the marketing budgets of the billion pound pharmaceutical industry. As a result most doctors are not as up to date with some of the excellent and effective principles of nutritional therapy as they could be.

More facts about the contraceptive pill and HRT

Oestrogens and progestogens are used in both the contraceptive pill and HRT preparations. Both types of drug are associated with water retention.

Other undesirable side-effects

At a conference held in London in 1997 by Doctors Against Sex Hormone Abuse (DASH), many of those attending said they were worried by the growing tendency to prescribe these drugs, partly because of their own experiences. Dr Margaret White described how she found it harder to come off HRT than to stop smoking. Dr Elizabeth Price developed severe side-effects when she used HRT and had to stop taking it. When she investigated the national statistics, she found that the suicide rate was twice as high in women taking HRT than in others. UK hospital admission rates are much higher among pill users than among those who use other contraception methods.

Most of the side-effects are mood disturbances, including aggression, depression and violence. According to a 1984 report by the British Royal College of General Practitioners, neurotic depression is the most common reason for women to come off the pill. Interactions between hormones and other drugs such as tranquillisers, caffeine and alcohol can make side-effects worse.

Dr Ellen Grant reported that, while it was once thought that only oestrogen increased the risk of thrombosis and heart attacks among pill users, it is now known that women over thirty-five who smoke and take contraceptives containing progestogens are 400 times more likely to have a heart attack than those who do not take the pill.

Professor Michael Steel looked at more than 75 studies linking the pill with breast cancer. Women who start taking the pill at an early age and continue taking it for a long time are four times more likely to get this disease. Out of every 100 women who use oestrogen-only HRT for ten years, one will develop breast cancer. Out of every 100 women who use combined oestrogen-progesterone HRT for ten years, two will develop it. Professor Steel said claims that taking the pill reduces the risk of ovarian cancer by 30–40 per cent are not borne out.

Professor James Walker reminded the audience that the synthetic oestrogen diethylstilboestrol (DES) was at first marketed as totally safe and given to 4.8 million pregnant women in the USA. Eventually found to be ineffective, it was banned in 1971.

Twenty years later, vaginal cancers were being discovered in daughters of the women who took DES. Many progestogens are derivatives of the male hormone testosterone and can have masculinising side-effects, he says.

Drug databases also report the following side-effects:

- Oestrogen-containing contraceptive pills can cause a deficiency of the B vitamin folic acid. Folic acid deficiency makes you more prone to heart disease and Alzheimer's disease, and can cause birth defects.
- If you are taking oestrogen and develop sudden severe tummy pain there is a possibility you may have a liver tumour.

Taking oestrogen can:

- Make you more likely to develop vaginal thrush (yeast infections).
- Change the surface of your eyes, causing problems with wearing contact lenses.
- Cause breast changes, including tenderness and enlargement.
- Increase your risk of stroke, heart attack, gall bladder disease, birth defects in your children, disturbances in vision, cancers and high blood pressure.
- Cause irregular brown patches to develop on your face within one month to two years. These may be permanent.

Taking progestogens can:

- Cause bleeding and spotting between periods.
- Cause severe depression.
- Increase your risk of heart attack, stroke, high blood pressure and embolism of the eyes (eye damage due to small blood clots).

- Cause headaches, nervousness, hair loss and changes in sex drive.

Coming off HRT

If you are on HRT and decide to stop taking it, you should do so under your doctor's supervision. Most women find that due to withdrawal symptoms it is best to reduce the HRT dose very gradually over about a year. One good method is to start by taking the patches off your skin for an hour or two each day, gradually building up the amount of time you spend without them. In the meantime, following the Waterfall Diet will help your body balance its own hormones, especially if you eat a lot of soya products such as soya milk, tofu and soya flour. In Japan, where women eat rice and soya every day, there is no word for 'hot flushes' because they are so rare!

If you are taking HRT to prevent osteoporosis, you may be interested to know that at least three medical journals have now reported that one of the most effective ways to prevent – and even reverse – osteoporosis is to consume foods and supplements rich in many minerals, especially magnesium and zinc, which are just as important as calcium and even more likely to be depleted in the average diet. Regular exercise like walking, swimming and trampolining is also very effective.

CHAPTER 6

How polluted are you?: Your body may be using water to dilute toxins

Two main types of water retention can be caused by internal pollution – high levels of substances that should not be there. The first type is cellulite, while the second is related to inflammation and leakage of your blood vessels, known in its most extreme form as vasculitis. This chapter looks at how internal pollution promotes cellulite and how to get rid of it naturally. It also describes how your liver works and advises on measures you can take to help your liver process toxins.

Case report: Elaine: 'Who says there's no such thing as cellulite?'

Elaine had been on every kind of diet, but while the rest of her grew thin and lissom, her thighs remained fat and lumpy with cellulite. Exercise made no difference. She was sceptical about the Waterfall Diet, but I explained that she had to use it together with vigorous massage for 8 minutes a day. 'Treat your thighs like bread dough,' I told her. 'Knead, pummel and squeeze them as much as you can to separate the fluid from the fat. Then the diet will help you get rid of both.'

Ten weeks later, Elaine's thighs measured 2 inches (5 cm) less in circumference and were getting into proportion with the rest of her body.

Internal pollution questionnaire

- Have you noticed an increasing tendency to feel tired most of the time?
- Do you get symptoms such as headaches, drowsiness, coughing or wheezing when exposed to fumes or chemicals such as dry cleaning or paint fumes, car exhausts, smoke, perfumes, cosmetics or household aerosols and sprays?
- Have you recently started to develop food allergies when you had none before?
- Have you been diagnosed with any of these illnesses?

  Alzheimer's disease
  arthritis
  asthma
  chronic fatigue syndrome
  kidney disease
  motor neurone disease
  Parkinson's disease
  psoriasis

- Do you appear to be ageing faster than other people of a similar age?
- Do you normally suffer from a tendency to constipation?
- Do you drink coffee several times a day?
- Do you smoke?

- Are you a medium to heavy drinker of alcohol?
- Do you have a lot of amalgam (silver) fillings?
- Do you regularly take medications – even if only aspirin, paracetamol (acetaminophen in the US) or the contraceptive pill?
- Do you consume a lot of processed foods or drinks containing artificial colourings, preservatives and other additives (e.g. dark brown beers, coloured soft drinks or sweets)? If you aren't sure, read the labels: the more words you don't recognise, the more of these undesirable substances are probably present.
- Do you eat less than two portions of fresh fruit or vegetables a day?

If you answered 'yes' to seven or more of the questions above, there is a strong likelihood that your water retention may be caused by internal pollution.

Cellulite

Cellulite can present a big weight problem. It is a type of body fat found almost exclusively in women and has a lumpy, dimpled appearance. It tends to collect around the thighs and is very hard to shift. The medical profession has divided views about it. Most doctors tell you that it doesn't exist, that it is no different from normal fat and can be lost by dieting and exercising. Some doctors' ears are closed to the women who tell them that this approach simply doesn't work. The doctors who do have treatments to offer are plastic surgeons, and they recommend liposuction: physically extracting the offending fat. Cellulite, they confirm, is a type of fat found deep in the skin. Its lumpy appearance is due to the uneven distribution of connective tissue below the skin in women – and it does not always respond to normal dieting and exercise.

What makes it different?

So far, the only explanation for why cellulite may not burn off like other fat comes from the world of natural medicine. The theory goes like this.

First, we know that only women get cellulite. Second, we know that a combination of a low-calorie diet with a 'cleansing' regime and plenty of vigorous massage can in time get rid of even the most resistant cellulite when ordinary dieting and exercise cannot. Third, we know that a number of toxic substances such as pesticides which we take in through food, air and water dissolve only in fat and not in water. These toxins cannot be excreted by your kidneys and if not properly broken down by your liver will tend to accumulate in your body fat. We also know that the ability of people's livers to break down these toxins and eliminate them from the body can vary sixty-fold, so some people will accumulate far more toxins in their body fat than others.

Natural medicine practitioners believe that female hormones somehow cause a woman's body fat to attract water when it is loaded with toxins. This water seems to prevent the fat from being broken down for fuel. When fat breaks down it releases toxins that are dissolved in it. These may travel to a woman's reproductive organs, damage her eggs or compromise a pregnancy. So cellulite may in fact be the body's deliberate way of encapsulating toxins to keep them safely out of harm's way.

The simple way to deal with cellulite

These are the four main parts of the anti-cellulite programme:

1. Vigorous massage of the affected areas for 8 minutes a day.
2. Follow the Waterfall Diet.
3. Take herbs and drink herbal teas which assist your liver and gall bladder.
4. Prevent constipation.

Vigorous physical pummelling, kneading and squeezing helps to separate the water from the fat in cellulite. You can then excrete the water and start to burn off the fat as fuel. But it's important to ensure that when toxins are released from the fat they don't just circulate around and then go back into storage, otherwise the problem would just start all over again. This is where the Waterfall Diet comes in. The Waterfall Diet encourages your liver to break down these toxins so that your body can eliminate them permanently.

Waste exits from your liver into your gall bladder and should then be released into your intestines, which carry it out of the body. If your gall bladder becomes stagnated from eating the wrong kind of food, it cannot do its job properly. Several foods, herbs, spices and herbal teas are very good at helping to stimulate the gall bladder. These are:

artichokes
beetroot and radish juice
turmeric (yellow Indian spice)
milk thistle (herb)
peppermint tea
dandelion coffee

It's also important to avoid constipation while treating cellulite. Toxins and wastes in your intestinal contents can be reabsorbed if they have to hang around too long because you are constipated.

Author Liz Hodgkinson has written books describing how it took her only about 12 weeks to rid herself of a severe case of cellulite by following these simple guidelines. She found that the most important part of her treatment was about 8 minutes of vigorous massage and pummelling of the problem areas every day. This is certainly worth trying before you opt for liposuction!

If this theory is one day proved, it will mean that cellulite is just another form of water retention. If, like many women, you want to urinate after massaging your problem areas for 8 minutes, you have probably released some retained fluid. Try measuring the circumference of your thighs after each massage. You may not get a noticeable difference for a while, but for research purposes I would love to know the results, so please do contact me via my website (www.health-diets.net). The fact that cellulite can sometimes be painful if you pinch it also suggests that it may be swollen with retained water.

Of course, even 'dimpled fat' sometimes does respond to dieting and exercise. I would like to propose that the more waterlogged it is, the less well it responds. Unfortunately, it is impossible to guess how much water is contained in cellulite just by looking at it.

Anti-cellulite herbs and other products

In 1999, a clinical trial was carried out in Australia on a natural anti-cellulite product called Cellasene. Based on the herbs ginkgo biloba and clover, plus evening primrose oil, fish oil and lecithin, the product was found effective by half the women who tested it.

Other natural health products said to aid cellulite reduction include aromatherapy oil mixtures which are applied to the skin during massage and are designed to stimulate the circulation in the area being massaged. Improved circulation helps to carry the retained fluid away from the area. Anything which helps to bring a warm glow to the cellulite area will be useful, so one ingredient of these products may be tiny amounts of pepper oil.

Other products are taken by mouth. These are likely to contain a lot of flavonoids – a type of nutrient found in fruit and vegetables – for instance blueberries, or the white pith of oranges and lemons. As we shall see in Chapter 8, a diet low in flavonoids is one of the commonest causes of water retention. The herb ginkgo biloba, which is an ingredient of Cellasene, is both rich in flavonoids and has been found in many clinical trials to improve circulation in the smallest blood vessels.

Clover flowers are traditionally known as a tonic for the veins and are rich in coumarins, one of the most effective nutrients for reducing Type II water retention. There will be more on this in Chapter 7.

Fucus vesiculosis, the seaweed bladderwrack, is added to some anti-cellulite products because of its iodine content. It is not specifically effective against cellulite, but a slight iodine deficiency in your diet can slow your metabolism, raise your oestrogen levels and make you gain weight. Iodine is vital for the proper functioning of the thyroid gland. People suffering from thyroid deficiency retain water in the tissues under their skin, which develops a puffy, waxy appearance. As reported as long ago as 1978 in the medical journal *Clinical Endocrinonology*, doctors don't always diagnose a thyroid deficiency soon enough. In this report, the Renal Research Laboratories at the North Staffordshire Medical Institute in England found that out of eleven of their patients with water retention, six had antibodies to their thyroid gland, meaning that this gland was damaged. When given thyroid hormone supplements, these patients lost their water retention. Yet according to standard medical tests, all the patients had normal thyroid glands. Clearly the normal tests were not sensitive enough. If you have had normal thyroid test results yet have any reason to suspect that you might be hypothyroid, it is worth bullying your doctor to send you for thyroid antibody tests. Alternatively, if you visit my website (www.health-diets.net), a test can be arranged for you there.

So-called 'liver' herbs, such as blue flag or dandelion root are sometimes added to anti-cellulite tablets because they help to drain the liver and gall bladder. This helps to prevent these wastes from going back into storage in your body fat.

Finally, one herb, *Centella asiatica* or gotu kola, has undergone some clinical trials on its own for the treatment of cellulite. In one trial, carried out by Dr A. Dalloz Bourguinon in 1975, a patient lost 5½ inches (14 cm) from the circumference of her thighs after using gotu kola together with a low-calorie diet for 55 days. But the average reduction in thigh circumference for the group of women as a whole was only 1 inch (2½ cm) during this time, and it is not known whether this might have been achieved with the diet alone.

Gotu kola (which is not related to the kola nut) is found in India, Australia, parts of Africa and the Far East. It is a source of therapeutic compounds and flavonoids, and has been used as a medicinal herb in India since prehistoric times, and also in Indonesia, mainly to aid the healing of wounds and to treat leprosy. In China it is favoured as an 'elixir of life' – a herb which promotes long life.

Scientists are interested in the therapeutic benefits of gotu kola, and several medical journals have reported the results of Italian researchers that extracts from this herb act as a skin and blood vessel strengthener and can treat leaky capillaries, varicose veins and chronic venous insufficiency – a condition where the legs swell up because the veins in the legs have difficulty in carrying the blood upwards against the flow of gravity.

Sensitivity to chemicals

You may have wondered why the questionnaire on page 69 asks whether you are sensitive to chemicals such as car exhausts, dry cleaning fumes, cigarette smoke or perfume. Chemical sensitivity is usually an indicator that the liver is overloaded with internal pollution and that you are at risk of developing water retention.

Doctors who specialise in environmental medicine carry out tests to see whether individuals with long-term health problems could be ill because they are sensitive to chemicals in food, air or water. These doctors carry out tests on the patient's liver, as a sluggish liver can lead to higher levels of internal pollution and greater sensitivity to chemicals. Examples of environmental illnesses are exhaustion, asthma or mental symptoms caused by breathing in fumes from paint, tobacco smoke, exhaust fumes, detergents or other household chemicals. (*For more on chemicals in the environment, see pp.78–9*).

The liver carries out its work by means of enzymes. These are substances produced by the body, which help to convert one chemical into another. Each enzyme does a specific job. In order to make enzymes, the body needs adequate amounts of nutrients such as vitamins, minerals and amino acids.

If the environmental doctor's tests identify a liver enzyme deficiency, the patient can be given extra amounts of the nutrients needed to make that enzyme. Together with a diet low in stressful foods, and a regime which reduces chemicals in the household, seemingly hopeless cases can be cured. Some of the illnesses which have been cured using these methods include vasculitis, asthma, severe chronic fatigue, Gulf War syndrome and autoimmune diseases such as rheumatoid arthritis. Vasculitis means inflammation of the blood vessels, and one of its symptoms is recurrent water retention. (Others are bruising and red marks around the affected vessels.) Autoimmune diseases are illnesses in which the cells of the immune system mistake the body's own organs and tissues for foreign matter and mount a destructive inflammatory attack against them. Inflammation causes swelling and water retention.

Success with treating vasculitis

One of the greatest environmental doctors today, Dr William Rea from Dallas, carried out a very interesting research study in 1976 on ten vasculitis sufferers. Dr Rea recorded all these patients' symptoms, looking for signs of allergy and chemical sensitivity. Apart from their vasculitis symptoms, all the patients also suffered from a stuffy nose and were very sensitive to cold. Most had muscle pains, sinusitis and regular headaches. Half had episodes of overwhelming fatigue and sore throats. Some also suffered from asthma, depression and cystitis. Most had had these illnesses for about twenty years and had seen at least ten doctors before consulting Dr Rea.

Dr Rea reasoned that since so many of these problems can be symptoms of allergic illness or chemical sensitivity, perhaps the vasculitis was too. He put the patients into a controlled environment where they could be kept away from all modern chemicals and stopped all their food and medications for a few days.

It took only four or five days for all the patients' symptoms to clear. Then they were 'challenged' with foods, tap water and the usual variety of everyday chemicals to which most of us are exposed: formaldehyde gas from soft furnishings, cigarette smoke, natural gas, chlorine and so on. The vasculitis and water retention reappeared in every case when small amounts of these chemicals were inhaled.

The effect of chemicals on your blood vessels

How could inhaling or consuming small amounts of chemicals cause inflammation of the blood vessels, bruising, swelling and water retention? Inflammation is triggered by the immune system, usually in response to a bacterial infection or an allergy. At the time of this research, Dr Rea did not know the answer, but he did know that bruising meant that tiny blood capillaries were being ruptured.

The answer may lie in the work of Dr John Gerrard, Professor of Pediatrics at the University of Saskatchewan in Canada. In his book *Food Allergy: New Perspectives* (Charles C. Thomas Pub. Ltd, 1980), he writes that the walls of blood vessels have an affinity 15 times greater than the rest of the body for phenol – a common type of toxic chemical used in plastic, among other things. This means phenols will tend to collect in and incorporate themselves into blood vessel walls. But if they do, will the cells of the vessel walls still look normal to your immune system? Or will they begin to look foreign and trigger an autoimmune attack? Many other chemicals such as formaldehyde, PVC and acetone have been shown to trigger pain and inflammation in blood vessels.

Vasculitis can also be triggered by a type of tissue damage called cross-linking, which can be caused by toxic chemicals and makes the wrong amino acids join up with each other. Cross-linking is destructive in many ways and accelerates the ageing process.

Source of chemicals in the environment

There are 60,000 chemicals in current commercial production. Three thousand of these are used as food additives and 800 are found in drinking water. All can contribute to your internal pollution. Pollutants can be absorbed from:

- Traffic fumes, especially carcinogenic particles in diesel smoke and lead from petrol.
- Factory and power station discharges into air, rivers and seas.
- Fish caught in polluted waters, especially in coastal areas.
- Food contaminated with pesticides.
- Industrial fallout (particles which were originally in fumes or smoke and have subsequently settled on crops and livestock).
- Invisible clouds of pesticide which can be blown halfway across the world. Pesticide is sprayed on pavements and parks, used in gardens, contained in wood preservatives, used on footpaths, road margins and in buildings. It is washed into the water table which provides our drinking water.

We can also bring pollution into our own homes by the products and services we use:

artificial air fresheners
artificial food additives
cosmetic aerosols and sprays, e.g. deodorant, hairspray, perfume
dry cleaning fumes
dust
fly spray and other insecticides
formaldehyde gas released by new carpets and furnishings
fumes from garages built underneath bedrooms or adjacent to living quarters
fumes from gas cookers and central heating

garden sprays

household sprays

mould from damp surroundings

re-used cooking oil (increases levels of harmful peroxides in food)

soap powders and detergents made from strong chemicals

strong-smelling fabric conditioners

strong-smelling polishes, toilet cleaners and carpet cleaners

tobacco smoke

unnecessary medications or recreational drugs

wood preservative

The body can also become polluted by toxins produced by an imbalance of bacteria in the intestines. This can lead to symptoms such as severe fatigue, bloating, headaches and foggy thinking.

How efficient is your liver?

To help prevent water retention caused by internal pollution, it is worth knowing a little bit about your liver, which has the job of keeping down your internal pollution levels. Some livers are better at this job than others. We have already mentioned that the ability of different people's livers to detoxify pesticides and other toxic substances can vary as much as sixty-fold. This means that one person who smokes sixty cigarettes a day and whose liver is very efficient at detoxifying the cancer-causing substances in cigarette smoke may be no more likely to get cancer than another who smokes only one cigarette a day, or even one who is only a passive smoker but has a particularly sluggish liver. The problem is that we have no way of knowing how efficient our liver is before we start smoking or before we realise that environmental toxins are affecting our health. We may have no idea that our liver is letting us down until we notice signs of 'internal pollution'. Have another look at the questionnaire on *p.69* to remind yourself of some of these signs and the ways you may be placing an extra burden on your liver and perhaps encouraging cellulite or vasculitis.

Dr Jean Monro of the Breakspear Hospital in the UK, who specialises in the treatment of people with illnesses caused by chemical sensitivity, has found that the livers of up to 58 per cent of her patients have difficulty in processing even mildly toxic substances like caffeine. As we shall see later, these livers are not diseased, but overworked and undernourished. Giving them more of the nutrients they need can in time help them to function better.

If you suffer from cellulite, vasculitis or any related water retention caused by internal pollution, your liver will need all the help you can give it. Do remember that your liver is completely dependent on you to look after it. Love your liver!

How your liver works

Many of the waste products found in your blood, as well as toxins ingested in your food, air and water, or as drugs and medicines, cannot be directly excreted by your kidneys. This is because they do not dissolve in water. Your liver's job is to take these toxins and change them until they do dissolve in water and so can be excreted in your urine. If that is not possible then your liver will send them to your gall bladder, to be excreted via your intestines. This process is usually known as 'detoxification', but more correctly as 'biotransformation' – the transforming of one substance into another, more excretable one (*see diagram on p.83*).

Liver detox: Phase I
There are two main phases of liver biotransformation. In Phase I, unwanted chemicals are made to undergo chemical reactions such as combining them with oxygen. Antioxidant vitamins such as vitamins C and E are used up in the process.

Eventually, step by step, liver enzymes turn the chemicals into intermediates, and then into acids. These acids are water-soluble, so your kidneys can excrete them.

As your liver acts on the unwanted chemicals, they don't necessarily get less and less toxic through the various stages. In fact, the intermediate chemicals created during Phase I can sometimes be a lot more toxic than the original ones. Cigarette smoke is an example. The bigger your liver's workload, the more toxic intermediate products will be made and the more antioxidant vitamins you need to process them. It may surprise you to know that smokers use vitamin C twice as fast as other people. Because their liver is coping with so much extra toxicity, they need to consume twice as much vitamin C as non-smokers just to maintain the same amount of this protective nutrient in their blood.

The names of some of the harmful intermediate toxins include:

free radicals
aldehydes
epoxides
chloral hydrate (identical to the knock-out drops known as the 'Mickey Finn')
Valium-like compounds.

Some of the well-known chemicals which have to go through Phase I biotransformation by your liver include:

caffeine
alcohol
dioxin (a pollutant)
exhaust fumes
organophosphorous pesticides
paint fumes
steroid hormones

drugs including paracetamol (acetaminophen), diazepam tranquillisers and sleeping pills, the contraceptive pill and cortisone.

The more of these you ingest, the more Phase I enzymes your liver
must produce, and the more antioxidants you must consume to
process them.

Liver overload

But what happens if for some reason there aren't enough enzymes
and antioxidants to go round?

Basically, the Phase I process will stop somewhere along the line.
The intermediate chemicals: free radicals, aldehydes, epoxides, chloral hydrate and Valium-like compounds will begin to build up. Can
you guess how these substances will make you feel as their levels
rise? People with a sluggish liver have reported feeling 'hung-over'
all the time, or drowsy, or suffering from depression and irritability,
water retention, problems with concentrating or fatigue. Often
people feel all right for most of the time, but exposure to fumes or
chemicals can tip the balance, bringing back the symptoms.

If you have this kind of chemical sensitivity, it can spread so that
an increasing number of chemicals could begin to affect you.
Eventually, you may even start reacting to the natural chemicals in
food and drink, such as natural insecticides in plants and ammonia
from consuming protein. If you come to associate your symptoms
with eating particular foods, you may believe that you have a food
intolerance (as described in Chapter 2), but in fact the symptoms are
a warning sign that your liver is overloaded.

The difference between a food intolerance and a sensitivity to the
natural chemicals in food is that in most cases of food intolerance
only one or two foods will make you feel ill. With a chemical sensitivity, on the other hand, you feel ill most of the time, because it
is virtually impossible to avoid all the common chemicals with
which we are surrounded.

If your liver is overloaded, the symptoms you experience depend

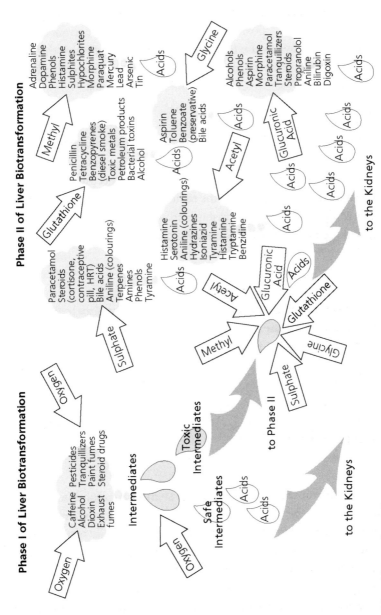

Liver biotransformation

on which type of intermediate chemical is building up in your system. Free radicals cause cells to die by rupturing their delicate protective outer membranes. Epoxides damage brain cells and increase the risk of cancer. Aldehydes (also found in cheap wine) cause headaches and, in severe cases, protein cross-linking and inflammation of the blood vessels or even epilepsy. Chloral hydrate and Valium-like compounds affect your concentration and can make you feel tired or drowsy.

As the immune system is activated in the parts of the body harbouring these chemicals, secondary reactions involving histamine and inflammation occur, and vary from person to person. Depending on where they become concentrated, they can cause anything from migraine to arthritis, asthma, vasculitis, water retention or skin reactions with rashes and swellings.

If this pattern of very poor health sounds like you, your liver may be in need of a helping hand.

Liver detox: Phase II

Phase II of the liver's detoxification work involves combining unwanted chemicals with one of five main types of substances that are found naturally in the body:

sulphate
acetyl groups
methyl groups
glucuronic acid
amino acids

The goal is still the same: to make the chemicals dissolve in water so that they can be excreted by the kidneys. Different chemicals are processed in different ways. So while caffeine is fully broken down by Phase I, paracetamol (acetaminophen) has to be combined with sulphate, and aspirin with glycine in Phase II.

Excessive internal pollution may be an explanation for the modern plague of chronic illnesses. Work carried out in recent years in England at Birmingham University by Dr Guy Steventon and Dr Rosemary Waring has shown that the livers of many people with chronic fatigue syndrome, Parkinsonism, motor neurone disease (also known as ALS) and Alzheimer's disease are more sluggish than those of healthy people in dealing with internal pollution. Similar work has been carried out at the University of Cincinnati in relation to bladder cancer. All this research has been published in several medical journals, including *Nature* and the *Lancet*.

Giving your liver a helping hand

If all this sounds rather daunting, don't worry! This book has not just been written for people with water retention who feel relatively healthy. Some individuals with this problem are quite poorly and will identify with and be greatly helped by the information in this chapter. Even if you are relatively healthy, I hope you will find these insights into liver overload interesting and that they will inspire you to work towards a healthier lifestyle.

The Waterfall Diet is a lifestyle change *par excellence* which can not only help your water retention but increase your chances of living an active, happy old age rather than the average old age, fraught with disabilities, that is suffered by so many. It really is never too late to start. If your liver is a bit sluggish, the Waterfall Diet can help it. Some care and attention and extra nutrients can make all the difference.

Eat the right foods
We can help our liver by eating foods which:

- Keep to a minimum the amount of unwanted chemicals.
- Nourish the biotransformation enzymes.
- Are rich in antioxidants.
- Provide abundant raw materials for Phase II.
- Help to stimulate the gall bladder.
- Help to prevent constipation.

The Waterfall Diet has been designed with this in mind and the appropriate foods are listed in the table below.

Avoid getting constipated

Foods high in dietary fibre are especially important for preventing one of the causes of internal pollution – constipation. Generally speaking, fibre is the indigestible part of our food, such as bran, cellulose and tough vegetable fibres and skins. Gum-like substances found in beans and seeds, and pectin, which is found in fruit, are also classified as dietary fibre. Fibre can absorb several times its weight in water and so it softens the stools and adds bulk. Your large intestine, or colon, needs this softness and bulk in order to move its contents towards the rectum, from which they can be evacuated.

Foods and nutrients which help biotransformation

Foods

brassica vegetables (broccoli, cauliflower, Brussels sprouts, cabbage)
dietary fibre
gelatine
protein

Vitamins

beta carotene
pantothenic acid (vitamin B5)
vitamin C
vitamin E

Minerals

magnesium
manganese
molybdenum

selenium
sulphate (found in Glauber's salts)

Amino acids
methionine
n-acetyl cysteine (NAC)
reduced glutathione
taurine

Herbs and spices which can help with liver protection and repair
milk thistle (herb)
turmeric (yellow Indian spice)

Herbs and drinks which can assist liver drainage
beetroot juice
dandelion coffee
golden seal (herb)
milk thistle (herb)
onions
radish juice
watercress

Besides fibre and water, your stools contain waste products excreted by your liver, toxins produced by the many bacteria which reside in your intestine and millions of dead bacteria. As this mixture of substances, known as faeces, enters your colon, it is quite liquid. One of the colon's jobs is to extract water from the faeces and to return it to the bloodstream, together with substances dissolved in it. Your body is only interested in useful dissolved substances such as vitamins and mineral salts. Unfortunately harmful wastes and bacterial toxins can also be absorbed back into your blood along with the water. The longer it takes for your faeces to be expelled in a bowel motion, the more unwanted substances can be reabsorbed in this way. Then your liver has to cope with them all over again. So it's important to have a bowel movement every day.

The benefits of different foods

Bran may help you to have bowel motions, but should not be your only source of dietary fibre. Eating a wide variety of wholegrains, beans, lentils and fresh fruit and vegetables, as in the Waterfall Diet, is the healthiest way to get all the different types of dietary fibre that your bowels need. It will also ensure that you benefit from the huge variety of nutrients found in these foods. By nutrients I don't just mean vitamins, minerals, starches and proteins, but essential polyunsaturated oils, flavonoids, carotenes and sterols, all of which are now known to play important roles in maintaining good health and preventing diseases.

Of the vegetables, broccoli, cauliflower and cabbage help the liver with its biotransformation work, while beetroot, radishes and onions help to drain your liver by stimulating your gall bladder. Your gall bladder is a tiny storage organ under your liver, which receives waste from your liver and releases it into your intestines. Beetroot juice has been recommended by naturopaths for a hundred years for this beneficial effect.

Why not add the bright yellow culinary herb known as turmeric, often found in Indian curries, to your cooking for its protective effect on your liver cells?

The medicinal herb milk thistle also protects liver cells from damage and helps to regenerate the liver if any previous damage has occurred. Many research studies on milk thistle and its extract silymarin have now been carried out, with excellent results.

Will fasting help your liver?

Although some books on naturopathy still recommend fasting as a technique to 'cleanse' the liver, we now know more about the functioning of the liver. Fasting is useful to rest the digestive system when it is overstressed, but when you are not eating you have to burn off body fat which contains stored toxins. The faster your body fat is burned off, the faster these toxins are released into your blood. Then your liver tries to process them, but cannot do this without a supply of protein. So if you have any doubts about your liver, keep up your intake of protein, fruit and vegetables.

Are dietary supplements worth taking?

Environmental medicine experts make great use of dietary supplements to help with the liver's biotransformation processes. The nutrients most needed can be determined with special liver function tests that use a 'marker' substance like caffeine or aspirin to measure how well each part of the biotransformation process is working.

In these tests, you consume a precise quantity of the marker substance. When broken down by a normal liver, it should result within a few hours in the appearance of a particular chemical in your urine. A sample of your urine is collected at a specific time and the amounts of this chemical are measured. If they are found to be too low, then you are lacking certain liver enzymes.

Sometimes only one set of enzymes is faulty, sometimes several. All enzymes are dependent on a range of nutrients and can often be improved when your diet is improved. It may be possible to get the necessary improvement in liver function just by eating a better diet. On the other hand, some people with this problem already eat an excellent diet but are not absorbing their nutrients very well. Pollution of all types really does increase our need for many vitamins, minerals, amino acids and other nutrients. Also, sometimes the body has problems in creating the more complex nutrients which it must make itself, such as such as the amino acids taurine and glutathione, and the fatty acids GLA and EPA. Using supplements as an added precaution ensures that nothing is left to chance and is very unlikely to cause harm. (*See p.216 for advice on how to choose a suitable multivitamin/mineral formula.*)

CHAPTER 7

Your personal plumbing system: Looking after your blood and lymph vessels

This chapter explains the normal processes of fluid exchange between your blood vessels and your tissues, and what actually happens at this level when things go wrong. It also looks at two more important causes of water retention: leaky blood vessels and congestion of your lymphatic system, which helps to drain away excess fluid.

Case report: John's new job

John was a couch potato. Unemployed, he sat around at home all day or lay in bed, watching TV and reading the newspaper. In the evenings he would visit friends, or they would come to see him, and enjoy a few cans of beer sitting around watching TV. Occasionally he went to the pub. He did not play any sports or take any other form of exercise.

Needless to say, John was getting more and more overweight. But when he tried a low-calorie diet for a while, it didn't seem to make much difference. Then he got a job packing shelves in a supermarket and within days the weight was falling off him. His previous lack of activity had slowed down his lymphatic system so much that fluid was not properly draining out of his tissue spaces but was collecting and adding to his weight problem. Once he got a job, the extra exercise activated John's lymphatic system and the fluid was able to drain away.

Answer the following questionnaire to see whether your water retention is due to problems with your blood capillaries or lymphatic vessels.

Capillary and lymphatic questionnaire

- Do you eat fresh fruit or vegetables less than once a day?
- If you are a woman, do you suffer from heavy menstrual periods?
- Do you bruise easily?
- Do your feet swell so much that your shoes no longer fit?
- Do you suffer from broken capillaries or thread veins?
- Do you avoid physical exercise?
- Do you sit still for several hours every day, for instance watching TV?
- Are you bed- or wheelchair-bound?

If you answered 'yes' to two or more of the first five questions, there is a strong possibility that your water retention is caused by leaky blood vessels. If you answered yes to any of the last three questions, your water retention may be caused or aggravated by lymphatic congestion.

The 'pipework' of your body (1): The circulation of the blood

Imagine that the fluid system in your body is similar to the one in your home – with mains pipes taking the fluid to smaller pipes and then to outlets, and a drainage network to carry away the waste water. In your body, the mains pipes are known as arteries. They are large and carry oxygen-rich 'arterial' blood consisting of:

red and white blood cells
platelet cells to help with clotting
plasma, a clear, watery fluid which contains dissolved nutrients and other substances.

In your arteries, blood is a very bright red because it is loaded with oxygen from your lungs. As soon as arterial blood leaves your lungs, it goes straight to your heart, which pumps it through your body with great force. This force is needed to get the blood, with its oxygen and nutrients, to all parts of your body.

Arteries branch off into smaller and smaller versions of themselves. The tiniest branches of all – hardly visible to the naked eye – are called capillaries, and you have about 25,000 miles of them in your body! Your arterial capillaries take blood to your tissues – the 'fabric' of your body, which consists of many kinds of cells. Examples are heart tissue, liver tissue, skin tissue and muscle tissue. A cell is the smallest unit of living matter.

How capillaries nourish your cells

Using a controlled filter built into their walls, the arterial capillaries release water enriched with oxygen and nutrients into your tissue spaces – the gaps between your cells. Your cells are bathed in this fluid. They absorb the oxygen and nutrients and discharge carbon dioxide and other wastes into it.

When the fluid enters your tissue spaces it is called tissue fluid

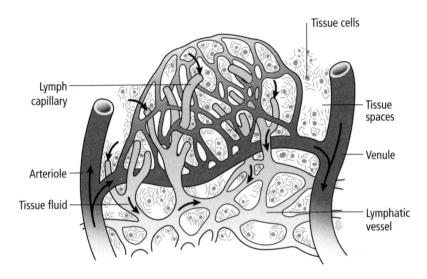

Lymph capillaries

or extracellular fluid. The tissue spaces have a very large capacity for holding fluid, and if you suffer from water retention this is the place where excess fluid builds up and collects.

As waste products from your cells collect in your tissue fluid, a reverse filter in your venous capillaries should suck the fluid back into your blood so that it can be taken away for processing. The venous capillaries link up to another set of large blood vessels, your veins, which take blood back to your heart.

Any excess fluid not removed from your tissue spaces by your venous capillaries is normally collected up and removed by your lymphatic system. This is a completely different network, which, as we shall see on page 99, plays a very important part in preventing water retention.

While the blood in arteries and arterial capillaries is bright red and full of oxygen and nutrients, the blood in your veins and venous capillaries is dark and full of waste products and carbon dioxide. The two blood systems are not separate; arterial capillaries eventually become venous capillaries, which then grow larger to become veins. Eventually the veins reach your heart, which pumps the blood to your lungs to pick up more oxygen and then back to your arteries again.

Your fluid balancing act

Your body tries to maintain a balance between the concentration of fluid in your blood and in your tissue spaces. So if your tissue fluid already contains a lot of glucose, your blood will hold on to its glucose instead of releasing it into the tissue spaces. On the other hand, if glucose is low in your tissue fluid, then your blood will quickly release some, until glucose concentrations are evenly balanced in both fluids.

This works in the other direction, too. Carbon dioxide can only get through to the blood if its levels are high in the tissue fluid. The same applies to water. Your body tries to keep the same levels of dilution and concentration in your blood and in your tissue spaces. When your tissue fluid is more saturated, your blood will send in more fluid to dilute it.

The volume of fluid in your tissue spaces should be three to four times greater than the volume of fluid in your blood, which is also known as your plasma. This balance depends on three factors:

1.   The concentrations of protein in your plasma and tissue fluid.
2.   The difference in fluid pressure on either side of your capillary walls.
3.   The 'leakiness' of your capillary walls.

The concentrations of fluid on either side of your capillary walls are correct when the blood pressure in your capillaries is low and protein levels are high. Your blood needs protein. We saw in Chapter 3 that an exceptionally low-protein diet can cause water retention. Without sufficient protein, your blood cannot draw water out of your tissue spaces.

Even when they eat plenty of protein, most people retain about 3 litres more fluid in their tissue spaces than their capillaries can re-absorb. So your tissue spaces need an 'overflow' system. It does indeed have one, and its name is the lymphatic system. We will give more information about this later in this chapter.

Water retention can also occur when the other balancing mecha-nisms are disturbed. Here's how they can go wrong.

Fluid pressure problems

Lots of things can interfere with the pressure on either side of your capillary walls. Hormones such as adrenaline (epinephrine), acetyl-choline and angiotensin can make your blood pressure go up or down by dilating or constricting small arteries. This happens when you are under stress, for instance. Adrenaline sends your blood pressure up by constricting the blood vessels at the outer edges of your body so that more blood is concentrated around your mus-cles, helping you to run away from, or fight, your source of stress.

In a healthy body, most pressure changes are only temporary and have no long-term effect on your tissue fluid. On the other hand, if your veins get blocked or congested, or your heart does not pump strongly enough, long-term pressure changes can reduce your abil-ity to reabsorb water from your tissue fluid. As we shall see, these situations can cause serious water retention and weight gain.

Congestive heart disease

This illness causes the severe water retention that used to be known as 'dropsy'. Poor pumping action by the heart reduces the flow of blood through the kidneys. This fools the body into think-ing that its total fluid levels are low rather than high, so it steps up its production of hormones to make the kidneys excrete less water. Urination diminishes, but blood fluid levels are in fact too high, not too low, so the excess fluid has to be sent for storage in the tissues.

In this condition, the feet and ankles are worst affected. The fluid pressure is greatest here because of the effects of gravity. Your feet and ankles can become so swollen that you need to wear support stockings and may have to buy shoes several sizes larger than usual.

If you have been diagnosed with this condition, your doctor has probably prescribed diuretic medicines to help stimulate your kidneys. A nutritionist can also advise you on natural remedies such as Coenzyme Q_{10}, which can usefully be added to the Waterfall Diet.

Leaky capillaries

Capillary walls should allow fluid and other substances to permeate through them into your tissue spaces. In a healthy person their permeability is strictly controlled. But if your capillary walls somehow become too 'leaky', too much protein as well as fluid can escape into your tissue spaces. This leads to a different type of

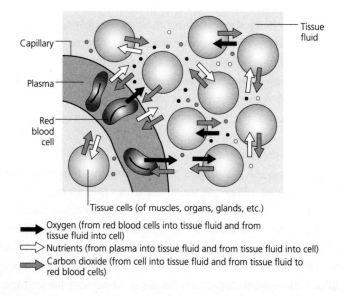

How substances are exchanged between capillaries, tissue fluid and cells

water retention, which I call 'Type II water retention'. Remember that protein attracts water? Well, if too much protein escapes from your blood into your tissues spaces, it is very hard for it to get back again. So it accumulates in your tissues spaces, where it attracts water. The more protein leaks out of your capillaries, the more fluid will shift from your blood into your tissue spaces. Your blood can even begin to get dehydrated, so your body tries to slow down urination. This of course worsens the water retention. To prevent Type II water retention, capillary health and strength is very important.

What makes capillary walls too leaky?
Several things can make your capillary walls more fragile or leaky:

- allergies and histamine
- shock
- infections
- damage to your capillaries by physical injury (e.g. bruising, friction or radiation)
- nutritional deficiencies which make your blood vessels more fragile
- imbalances in hormone-like substances known as prostaglandins (*see pp.121–2*).

An example of fluid leaking from damaged capillaries is the blister effect. Friction from a badly-fitting shoe, for instance, or heat from a burn, damages the capillaries under your skin. These leak fluid under the surface layer of your skin, forming a blister.

Histamine, a chemical released when allergic reactions occur, can have a similar damaging effect. It temporarily widens the joints between the cells that form your capillary walls, allowing fluid to leak out between them. Signs of leaky capillaries include a tendency to:

- Bruise too easily.
- Suffer extensively from thread (spider) veins or little red blood marks under the skin.
- In women, have heavy menstrual periods.

How to keep your capillaries in good condition

It is important to give your capillary walls enough nutrients to keep them strong and healthy. The nutrients they need most – vitamin C and flavonoids (*see p.124*) are found in fruit and vegetables. The white 'pithy' part of oranges is especially good, being very rich in flavonoids. Of course there are other causes of heavy menstrual periods besides leaky or fragile capillaries, but I have known several cases where women who had this problem cured it by improving their consumption of fresh fruits and vegetables. If you do not eat fresh fruit and vegetables every day, you could be at risk of water retention.

Flavonoids can also be taken as dietary supplements. In one scientific study carried out in France, flavonoid supplements were successfully used to treat fifteen cases of water retention caused by excessively leaky capillaries.

Treating damaged capillaries with flavonoids is not a new notion. In fact, the connection between flavonoids and capillary health has been known for 50 years. Several scientific studies in the 1950s found that capillary damage caused by radiation treatments could be much reduced by supplementing the diet with vitamin C and/or flavonoids. (*For more about capillaries, see p.106.*)

More about Type II water retention

As we know, leaky capillary walls can leak too much protein from your blood into your tissue spaces. The protein sits there, attracting water from your blood into your tissue spaces, which leads to water retention. I have termed this 'Type II' water retention because it requires a different treatment. This water cannot be reduced by taking diuretic medicines. In fact, by dehydrating your blood, diuretics could even make it worse.

Provided the amount of protein in the tissue fluid is not too great, all is not necessarily lost. Your lymphatic system can absorb some protein from your tissue fluid and return it to your blood – in fact this is a routine part of its work. Healthy capillaries do normally release a little bit of protein into your tissue fluid, and it is only when your lymphatics fail to drain it away that the protein levels in your tissue fluid will rise. The next section is all about keeping your lymphatic system as healthy as possible so that it can do its important job.

The 'pipework' of your body (2): The lymphatic system

Lymph vessels are present in almost every organ of the body, and are extremely important in preventing water retention. As we know, they help to drain away excess tissue fluid. Lymph vessels have very thin walls and large pores: they easily absorb tissue fluid and any proteins that it contains.

Once your tissue fluid enters your lymphatic system it is known as lymph and is channelled through your lymph vessels, which converge to form ever-larger vessels. The two largest drain into veins in your neck, thus returning fluid to your blood. If your lymphatic system gets blocked, you can develop severe water retention because tissue fluid will be unable to return to your blood.

Exercise is important for lymph vessels

Unlike your blood circulation, lymph has no heart to pump it around. Lymph will only flow if you move your body. When your muscles work, they massage your lymph vessels and stimulate the flow of lymph. So regular exercise is really important to combat water retention.

One reason why long-distance flights are known to cause water retention in feet and ankles is the fact that passengers have to sit in cramped conditions, virtually immobile, for hours on end. Likewise, complete bed-rest can cause devastating water retention, which hospital staff usually try to prevent by making patients get out of bed from time to time, even after major surgery. The modern couch potato lifestyle is responsible for a type of water retention which actually has a special medical name – it is known as 'television oedema'. Moving about helps to prevent the problem. Even if you only move your foot, the lymphatic vessels in your leg can work much more effectively than if your foot is completely still. So don't forget to keep wiggling your toes whenever you are on an aeroplane.

Massage is good too

If exercise is impossible, the next most effective way to stimulate your lymphatic circulation is with massage. This does not have to be vigorous. Your lymph vessels are delicate and can get damaged if you massage too hard. See the diagram on page 108 for the correct massage points and directions. One reason why we automatically massage ourselves when we have received a bump or bruise is because we unconsciously know that we need to stimulate the lymphatic system around the injured part in order to drain away the fluid released by injured capillaries.

Injuries can also develop water retention, which makes them more painful. When I was involved in a minor car accident I severely wrenched one of my fingers and suffered pain and swelling around one of the joints for nearly a year afterwards. Daily massage helped to drain away the fluid which was causing the painful pressure. The fact that it took so long for the swelling to go down is not unusual, according to lymphologists – doctors who specialise in disorders of the lymphatic system.

Water retention under the eyes, producing baggy lower eyelids, occurs when tissues are excessively compliant; that is to say, as they absorb more fluid, they expand too easily. So if you suffer from this problem, the delicate tissues under your eyes need a little assistance from you. All tissues can be weakened by a lack of vitamin C or by failure to consume enough flavonoids from fruit and vegetables, so the Waterfall Diet includes plenty of these nutrients. Daily gentle massage, not just around your eyes but of your face, neck and armpits too, will help your lymphatic system to drain. Do ensure as well that you get enough exercise, especially of your upper body – for instance, daily arm-swinging and head-rolling exercises.

Lymph nodes

Your lymph is filtered by lymph nodes positioned in your neck, armpits, groin, tummy and other places. If these nodes are removed by surgery, or if they become inflamed or hardened, your flow of lymph can become blocked. If this occurs in an arm or leg, that limb could become very swollen while the rest of your body remains normal.

All parts of your body are drained by your lymphatic system, and Dr Casley-Smith points out that diseases of almost every organ can be caused or greatly worsened by congestion of the lymphatic system. Even so-called autoimmune diseases, where your white blood cells attack your joints, nerve cells or thyroid gland, for instance, can be triggered when your immune system becomes overactive as a result of excess protein leaking from fragile capillaries into the tissue spaces.

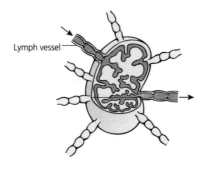

Lymph node

Complications of Type II water retention

Inflammation, such as caused by an injury, or from allergic reactions, is another cause of Type II water retention. But, because of the protein it contains, Type II water retention makes it difficult for the inflammation to heal itself. Accumulations of protein in the tissue spaces have an inflammatory effect, causing pain and swelling. So a sprain or other injury, for instance, can continue to be painful and swollen for years.

This area of research has been written about extensively by Dr John Casley-Smith, past President of the International Society for Lymphology, working at the University of Adelaide in Australia. In his medical book *High Protein Oedemas and the Benzo-pyrones*, he looks in depth at how inflammation can lead to Type II water retention.

Causes of inflammation

- Inflammation can start when blood vessels are injured by a blow, sprain, excessive friction or by chemical damage. For instance, a single severe exposure to an inhaled irritant like the weed-killer Paraquat has been known to cause long-term inflammation in the lungs, which gradually destroys them.
- Infections, and histamine from allergic reactions or irritation also cause inflammation.
- Long-term inflammation can occur after injuries or obstructions to the lymphatic system.
- Lack of exercise encourages inflammation by congesting the lymphatic system.

Inflammation widens the joints between the cells that form the capillary walls, allowing protein to leak out of the capillaries into the tissue spaces. This protein can prolong the inflammation if it is not broken down and drained away. Inflammation can become chronic or long-term when blood vessel walls damaged by nutritional deficiencies chronically leak too much protein-rich fluid into the tissues. Deficiencies of the vitamin B complex, vitamin C and the flavonoids are especially problematic.

What damage does long-term inflammation cause?

Long-term inflammation can start a vicious circle which begins with hardening the tissues so that lymphatic drainage becomes more difficult. This tends to worsen Type II water retention. For instance, someone with a sprained ankle may find that three years later their ankle is still swollen and painful, and shows no signs of getting better. The pain and swelling is no longer due to the original injury but to the tissue hardening (fibrosis) and lymphatic blockage which was caused by the inflammation.

Second, inflammation has a destructive effect on the tissues. The white blood cells which come to inflamed areas produce enzymes designed to break down the proteins which have leaked into the tissue spaces. These enzymes tend to break down the body's tissues too. In the short term these tissues can heal themselves, but when inflammation becomes chronic, they never get the chance. Gum disease – the main cause of tooth loss after the age of 30 – is a good example. As mouth bacteria settle into the tiny gaps between your teeth and gums, your white blood cells attack them, starting off an inflammatory process which makes your gums tender and bleed easily. If the bacteria are not removed by regular cleaning, this inflammation gradually deepens, and destroys the gums until the teeth become loose and drop out.

Another example is osteoarthritis, a disease where joints become swollen and cartilage is eaten away. This probably starts off as too much friction around the joint. Protein which has leaked from fragile, friction-damaged capillaries remains in the tissues around the joint instead of being drained away by the lymphatic system. Long-term low-grade inflammation eventually sets in, causing damage to the joint itself. There can be lots of reasons for the excessive friction which started it all off. One reason is failure to drink enough water. The cartilage which is designed to prevent friction in joints can dehydrate and shrink if you become dehydrated.

Chilblains which take a long time to heal and lead to enlarged, hardened finger joints are a good example of inflammation causing tissue hardening or fibrosis. Chilblains are probably caused by a combination of nutritional deficiencies which make blood capillaries too fragile and too easily injured and leaky when cold fingers or toes are placed too close to a fire or radiator.

Lung and eye problems

When the lymphatic drainage of your lungs is impaired, chronic bronchitis and emphysema – a disease in which inflammation progressively destroys the lungs – may result. Even your eyes can suffer from water retention. The disease known as macular degeneration – a common cause of blindness – is associated with pools of excess protein leaking from the capillaries behind the retina.

Water retention breaks vital contacts between cells

Another complication of water retention is the 'stretching' effect which excess fluid has on your tissue spaces. The more these spaces become engorged with fluid, the further away your cells become from their source of vital oxygen and nutrients and from each other. Even minor water retention can break the cell-to-cell contacts which assist the passage of oxygen from your capillaries to the part of the cell where it is needed.

As yet, we know very little about the effects this can have on your body. We know that when cells are starved of oxygen, wounds fail to heal properly, but when the nutrients in your tissue spaces are diluted by too much fluid, are your cells still able to absorb them properly?

A possible cancer risk

It is scientifically well established that when your tissue spaces become oversaturated with fluid, they also become much more permeable to all kinds of possibly toxic particles which they would not normally absorb. As harmful substances such as free radicals come into contact with your cells they can rupture the delicate membrane which covers them, damaging the cell and allowing genetic material to leak out.

As explained by Dr Nadya Coates in her book *A Matter of Life*, it is a law of life that every piece of genetic material 'wants' to become a cell and to become a nucleus, but cannot do so without the full genetic information required for a cell to reach proper maturity. Cancer starts when an incomplete cell begins to reproduce wildly. Normally your immune system will seek out and destroy such abnormal cells, but the various types of disruption which water retention and fibrosis bring to the affected areas – such as reducing the oxygen supply and blocking the passage of white cells – could cause the immune system to become less efficient at destroying cancer cells.

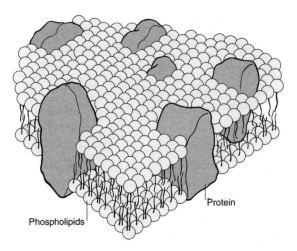

Protein

Phospholipids

Cell membrane

More facts about your capillaries

Your capillary network extends to almost every tissue of your body. Each capillary is about 1 mm long and none of the cells in your body should be more than 0.1 mm away from a capillary. Capillaries are so tiny they can hardly be seen with the naked eye. The capillary itself is a tube whose walls are made up of flat cells one layer thick. These, known as endothelial cells, fit together with narrow gaps or 'pores' between them. On the other side of the capillary wall is the tissue fluid, the watery fluid in your tissue spaces which bathes your cells. Oxygen and fat-soluble nutrients (nutrients which can dissolve in oil but not in water) pass from your blood through the endothelial cells to get to your tissue fluid. Water, glucose and other water-soluble nutrients pass through the pores in between. Once in the tissue fluid, these substances can be taken up as needed by your cells. Waste products such as carbon dioxide are released from your cells into your tissue fluid, and from here can pass into your capillaries ready for processing or elimination.

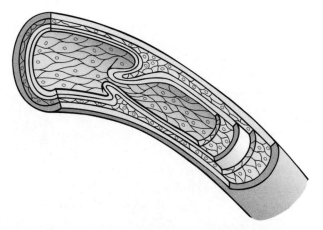

The walls of a vein, showing how the cells are arranged. In a capillary, fluid escapes through the 'seams' between the cells.

Improving lymphatic congestion

Don't be daunted by this information. It is only included to help you take seriously the kind of lifestyle changes which will help prevent health problems or worse water retention in later life.

Movement

To keep your lymphatic system healthy, avoid remaining immobile for many hours (e.g. watching television).

If you suffer an injury, don't let the pain keep you immobile. You don't need to move broken bones, but if you have a broken arm, for instance, you could rotate your head and shoulder a little from time to time, stretch the rest of your body and massage under your armpit. Even small, gentle movements like these help the lymphatic system to drain away the fluid which is pressing on the injury and making it more painful.

If you suffer from any type of paralysis, regular massage becomes all the more important. Chronic fatigue syndrome patients may find that getting someone to massage them every day may help some of the soreness that bed-bound sufferers often experience, which can be due to fluid build-up (*see p.108.*)

Choose flavonoids, not diuretics

It is important not to take diuretics for Type II water retention. They may appear to remove water, but they will dehydrate you, and the protein causing the water retention will quickly attract fluid back into your tissues. The dehydration will also constipate you, make you retain sodium and so aggravate your water retention. French kidney specialist Dr G. Lagrue says that water retention can be caused by abusing laxatives and diuretics.

Another medical treatment for Type II water retention is used by lymphologists in Australia, Germany and Italy. It consists of the flavonoids quercetin and rutin together with a plant extract known as coumarin (*see Chapter 8*). As mentioned in Chapter 6,

Lymph drainage massage

The right kind of massage can improve the flow of lymph. Start by gently massaging the neck, tummy, groin and armpit areas. This helps to empty the lymph nodes in these areas. Then massage the rest of the trunk, followed by the thighs and upper arms. Always stroke towards the centre of the body. Gradually extend the area of massage towards the hands and feet. Some popular books suggest using a dry brush on the skin, but this is harsh on the skin and it is not known whether it provides enough stimulation to help 'pump' the lymph along. Also, some of these books wrongly state that the brush strokes should have an outward direction.

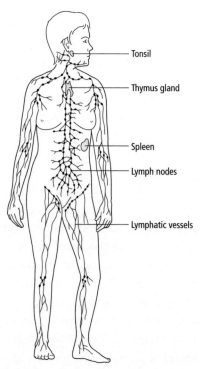

How to give yourself a lymph drainage massage

> Lympholgists recommend that athletes and dancers should practise lymph drainage massage whenever they get sprains or other mild injuries. A minute spent emptying the lymph nodes in the groin by massage, and making cycling movements with your feet in the air while lying on your back, can reduce pain in a sprained ankle and improve its mobility by reducing the swelling.

flavonoids are important nutrients in fruits and vegetables which help to keep blood vessels strong and prevent them from leaking. But Dr Casley-Smith has also carried out some fascinating research which shows that, given in very high doses, they can encourage the proliferation of the white blood cells known as macrophages, which gather in parts of the body affected by Type II water retention. These macrophages split the accumulated protein into small fragments. Once broken down into amino acids, the proteins are much more easily able to pass back through the capillary walls and back into the bloodstream.

If you suffer from varicose veins, you may be interested to know that one of the above-mentioned nutrients, rutin, helps to repair damage to elastin and collagen in the walls of your veins. We mentioned in Chapter 6 that the herb gotu kola can help varicose veins. Since herbs are plants which often contain the same flavonoids as foods, but perhaps in higher concentrations, it makes sense that some herbs work not by having a medicinal effect but by correcting long-term nutritional deficiencies.

CHAPTER 8

Water retention caused by vitamin and mineral deficiencies

It is perfectly possible to have symptoms of vitamin or mineral deficiencies even if you eat a healthy, nourishing, well-balanced diet.

Would you know if you had a nutritional deficiency? Not necessarily. A lot of the symptoms of vitamin and mineral deficiencies are things we easily take for granted:

bad skin
getting tired easily
not sleeping well
mood swings
bad nerves
period pains

As we already know, a protein deficiency can cause water retention, but good fluid balance also depends on adequate amounts of the so-called 'micronutrients': vitamins, minerals, essential fatty acids, flavonoids and so on. This chapter looks at some of the ways in which these nutrients can affect your fluid balance, how nutritional deficiencies occur and how you can tell if you have them.

Case report: Barbara needed zinc

Barbara consulted me when she was seven months pregnant. She was twenty-three and a vegetarian, and it was her first baby. She came somewhat reluctantly, at the instigation of her mother-in-law. Barbara's appetite was so poor that she ate foods only for their taste, not from hunger. While the rest of the family had a complete meal, she might pick at a piece of cheesecake.

Barbara was badly anaemic. Her haemoglobin levels had been progressively dropping since the early stages of pregnancy, despite increasing doses of iron prescribed by her doctor. By the time she consulted me her skin was extremely pale and the anaemia was causing severe water retention, particularly in her legs. The extra fluid was in turn pushing her blood pressure sky-high and both mother and baby were at risk. Barbara agreed to see me because her doctor wanted to keep her in hospital in order to give her iron injections. She had refused this and was desperately seeking alternatives.

The foods Barbara did eat included a lot of fatty foods, white bread, chocolate, crisps and biscuits. She had received counselling about iron-rich foods from a hospital dietician, but couldn't follow the advice because she had no appetite.

She told me that she suffered from permanent sores inside her nose and that during the first three months of her pregnancy she had felt nauseous twenty-four hours a day. In my opinion, these symptoms plus the anaemia and water retention pointed to severe zinc deficiency. Her diet excluded meat and fish, from which most people get their zinc, and was also lacking in wholegrains, which are a vegetarian's source of zinc. To make matters worse, iron supplements can interfere with the absorption of zinc from food – yet her doctor was prescribing very large amounts of iron.

After asking her to obtain her doctor's permission to stop the iron supplements, I gave Barbara multivitamins and minerals plus zinc, together with some counselling along the lines of the Waterfall Diet. To her doctor's amazement, Barbara's haemoglobin levels started to rise within days. She went on to produce a healthy baby.

Nutritional deficiency questionnaire

- Do you have white spots on your fingernails?
- Do you always seem to be getting colds or flu?
- Do you find it hard to grip pens, cutlery or tools?
- Do you accidentally drop and break things much more than you used to?
- You get a lot of twitches or spasms, or a flickering feeling in your eyelids?
- Do you feel like fainting if you miss a meal?
- Do you have a poor sense of taste or smell?
- Do you get a lot of palpitations and/or breathlessness from minor exertion?
- Is your sleep almost always dreamless?
- Are you always getting sores at the corners of your mouth or itchy red patches around eyebrows or behind ears?
- Is your tongue usually very red or shiny?
- If you are a woman, do you gain several pounds or experience a swollen tummy before your periods?
- If you are a woman who has reached the menopause, have you developed painful knots on the sides of your finger joints?
- Do you eat fresh fruit and vegetables less than once a day?
- Do you normally eat white bread rather than wholemeal?
- Do you put sugar in tea or coffee?
- Weight for weight, do you consume as much sugary food (e.g. sweets, chocolate, cakes, biscuits, jam, honey, syrup, ice cream,

sugary cereals, desserts and sweet drinks) as other foods – or perhaps even more?

- Do you eat fried or fatty food such as burgers, sausages or pastry every day?
- Has there ever been a time in your life when you ate an extremely poor diet for several months or even years?

If you have answered 'yes' to six or more of the above questions, your water retention could be due to nutritional deficiencies.

B_6 – an exciting discovery

Pyridoxine, or vitamin B_6, was isolated in 1938. It seems incredible that we have known about this important nutrient for such a short time, and even more incredible that only in 1952 was it found to be essential for human life. The discovery happened when some babies in the USA developed convulsions after consuming an over-cooked commercial milk formula. The cause of the convulsions was found to be a deficiency of vitamin B_6, which is destroyed by heat. A fascinating account of this discovery is given in a book published in 1973, *Vitamin B_6: The Doctor's Report*, by Dr John Ellis from Texas.

Dr Ellis developed a strong interest in vitamin B_6 in 1961, and spent the next nine years conducting clinical studies in its thera-peutic use. Around this time doctors were finding that more and more ailments responded to vitamin B_6 therapy, which of course implied that they had been brought on by a deficiency of this vita-min. These ailments included seizures in children with learning difficulties, neuritis from anti-TB drugs, nausea from cancer radio-therapy treatments, anaemia which did not respond to the usual therapies, and sunburn after very little exposure to the sun. Also, Dr Ellis found that vitamin B_6 deficiency could cause severe water retention.

The diet that worked

His interest began when he started to investigate diet and nutrition after heart disease had killed several of his patients. After reading about the Morrison diet, recommended in the *Journal of the American Medical Association*, he began prescribing it to his patients. The diet advocated lean instead of fatty meat, increased consumption of fresh fruit and vegetables, and the use of vegetable oils instead of animal fats.

Many of his patients had complained of tingling sensations, cramps and spasms, but the diet appeared to relieve these symptoms. Some patients whose hands were puffy (a sign of water retention) and could not bend their fingers very well lost both the puffiness and several pounds in weight, and became able to bend their fingers easily within a few weeks and without cutting down on their calorie intake. One of the patients had cured pains in his knees by eating pecan nuts every day and said that he too had lost stiffness in his fingers and now had a stronger grip. The doctor added pecan nuts to the Morrison diet and got even better results.

Putting two and two together

At this point, Dr Ellis didn't know why the diet was bringing these improvements, but he did know that it was much richer in B vitamins than the kind of food his patients had previously been eating. He persuaded some of them to try vitamin B injections for the tingling and pains in their hands, and he found this treatment to be just as successful as the new diet. Putting two and two together, he concluded that:

- The numbness, tingling, pains, puffiness and gripping problems were caused by water retention.
- The water retention was a symptom of B vitamin deficiency.

No doctor had ever reported this before.

The proof

Excited at his findings, Ellis wondered which specific B vitamin his patients most lacked. It could not be B_1, because this deficiency caused tremors of the tongue. B_2 deficiency led to little sores in the corners of the mouth. B_3 deficiency gave rise to dermatitis. His patients did not have any of these symptoms.

No medical reports had yet suggested that B_6 deficiency could occur in adults, but Dr Ellis wondered what the symptoms would be if it did. He decided to try injecting plain vitamin B_6 into his patients, knowing that, medically speaking, he was in completely uncharted territory. As he waited for the results, he knew he could be on the threshold of a tremendous discovery. Water retention was one of the most baffling problems facing his medical colleagues.

Seeing the first patient return to his surgery after four days, having lost so much excess fluid that her shoes were now several sizes too big for her, was the greatest thrill Dr Ellis had experienced in his entire medical career.

What are the symptoms of vitamin B_6 deficiency?

While official textbooks were slow in catching up with John Ellis' observational studies on his patients, they do now recognise that vitamin B_6 deficiency can occur in adults, particularly in those who drink a lot of alcohol and women who take the contraceptive pill.

They also recognise that, because people with vitamin B_6 deficiency excrete larger amounts of a chemical known as oxalate in their urine, they are at greater risk of developing kidney stones. Pregnancy, heart failure and radiation exposure are also recognised as leading to higher requirements for B_6. Experimental B_6 deprivation has brought symptoms of irritability, weakness, insomnia and poor coordination, say the official books. Nowhere is there any reference to water retention. Yet without vitamin B_6, important amino acids cannot be synthesised from other amino acids; the vital brain messenger chemicals serotonin, noradrena-line and histamine cannot be made from amino acids tryptophan, tyrosine and histidine. Vitamin B_3 cannot be made from tryptophan. Perhaps most important of all, vitamin B_6 assists in the transport of amino acids from the intestine across the gut wall and in the blood. Without this transport, a protein deficiency could develop.

Lymph expert Dr John Casley-Smith, whose work was men-tioned in Chapter 7, has something to say about water retention and the B vitamins. He points out that a diet lacking these nutri-ents causes the gaps between cells lining the capillaries to open up, allowing protein to escape into the tissue spaces, where it lies attracting fluid. And in experiments, rats deprived of all B vita-mins for 42 days develop leaks in their lymphatic vessels. Giving them vitamins B_5 or B_6 or flavonoids (*see p. 124*) prevents this. Diets lacking in flavonoids, or in vitamin C, can make capillaries even more leaky, and advanced vitamin C deficiency – the condition known as scurvy – leads to leakage of whole blood, not just fluid, out of the capillaries, so that you can even see little red blood marks under the skin.

Premenstrual syndrome (PMS)

Millions of women experience the discomfort of swollen, painful breasts and bloated tummies around the time of their period. These symptoms are due to water retention. If you suffer from them, you will probably have noticed that your body weight goes down soon after your period starts.

Writing in the *Journal of Reproductive Medicine* (1983), nutrition specialist Dr Guy Abrahams is sure that premenstrual water reten-tion is caused by temporary deficiencies of vitamin B_6 and the mineral magnesium, brought on by the heavy demands of hor-monal cycles. In a woman's monthly cycle, oestrogen levels steadily increase until ovulation, after which she makes more progesterone and her liver breaks down oestrogen. All these processes make heavy use of many nutrients. Since vitamin B_6 plays an especially important role, it risks getting depleted.

B_6 deficiency not only promotes water retention by weakening the capillary walls but can also affect your body's excretion of sodium. Both B_6 and the mineral magnesium are required to produce a hormone known as dopamine. Dopamine normally helps you to excrete sodium and water, and Dr Abrahams quotes research which has found that women who retain fluid premenstrually have lower dopamine levels.

Finally, vitamin B_6 and magnesium (among other nutrients) are needed for the production of beneficial prostaglandins, which are also involved in controlling the body's fluid balance. (*There is more about this on p.121.*)

Reports that B_6 supplements can prevent the symptoms of premenstrual syndrome have been published in the *Journal of International Medical Research* in 1985, the *Journal of Reproductive Medicine* in 1987, the *Lancet* in 1988 and the *British Medical Journal* in 1999, among others. But this has not led to them being used as a treatment, except by doctors who specialise in nutritional medicine. In view of the methods used in these studies, this is not really surprising. As we know, the causes of even such an apparently straightforward symptom as water retention can be complex and varied. So before giving a woman a vitamin B_6 supplement, it would make sense to test her first for B_6 deficiency. Sadly, this has not been done in PMS research studies.

Several hundred enzyme reactions in the human body depend on magnesium. But when doctors in the UK test for nutritional deficiencies, they find magnesium (and zinc and selenium) are lacking more frequently than any other minerals.

Magnesium deficiency

Most people eat a diet low in magnesium-rich foods such as wholemeal bread, oatmeal, nuts, sesame seeds and dark green leafy vegetables. Did you know, for instance, that white flour contains only one-third as much magnesium as wholemeal flour? To make matters worse, excessive protein in your diet, especially dairy produce, can reduce your body's absorption of magnesium because of the high phosphorus and calcium content. So a possible magnesium deficiency is further aggravated.

Coffee consumption increases the excretion of magnesium and other minerals. Magnesium can also be depleted by:

> chronic diarrhoea
> overuse of enemas or laxatives
> the contraceptive pill
> stress (one of the biggest drains on magnesium)

A little-known fact is that stress hormones such as adrenaline (epinephrine) and cortisol lower your body's magnesium levels. According to specialist researchers, all stress, whether exertion, heat, cold, trauma, pain, asthma attacks, anxiety or even excitement, can have this effect and so increase your need for magnesium. This important subject was extensively reviewed in 1994 in the prestigious *Journal of the American College of Nutrition*.

Since magnesium is needed for so many enzymes in your body, it is involved in fluid balance in many ways. For instance, it is known to biochemists that magnesium and potassium work so closely together in the body's cells that doctors cannot improve low potassium levels in their heart patients, for example, or in patients on potent diuretic drugs, unless they first correct any magnesium deficiency.

The journal *Archives of Internal Medicine* (1992) reports that 38–42 per cent of such patients have magnesium deficiency, and the *American Journal of Medicine* goes even further, stating that 'Hypomagnesemia [magnesium deficiency] is probably the most underdiagnosed electrolyte deficiency in current medical practice.' (*See Chapter 4 for information on electrolytes and their role in deciding how much water your kidneys should excrete.*) If you are retaining fluid because you are losing too much potassium, it may be because you are lacking magnesium, and so you may benefit by eating more magnesium-rich foods – as in the Waterfall Diet – and if necessary also taking magnesium supplements.

B$_6$ to the rescue

Vitamin B$_6$ helps to get magnesium across the cell membrane and into your cells. In one research study, published in the *Annals of Clinical Laboratory Science* (1981), a group of nine women were found to have low levels of magnesium in their red blood cells (magnesium deficiency shows up more quickly in the red blood cells than it does in the plasma, where it is usually measured). After they had received 100 mg of vitamin B$_6$ twice a day, these levels rose significantly and after four weeks of treatment they had doubled. If we make the reasonable assumption that red blood cells will only absorb as much magnesium as they need, this research suggests that these women's red cells were previously not absorbing enough magnesium due to a lack of vitamin B$_6$.

Yet more effects of magnesium deficiency

We have already mentioned that a magnesium (and B$_6$) deficiency reduces levels of dopamine, a hormone which aids urination. But according to research at the City of Hope Medical Center in Duarte, California (1993), a magnesium deficiency also raises levels of aldosterone, a hormone which slows down urination. So magnesium deficiency is a double candidate for promoting water retention.

High blood pressure caused by water retention in pregnancy (also known as pre-eclampsia) is now becoming recognised and treated as a magnesium deficiency condition. Magnesium treatments have proved to be more effective than drugs. It is very unfortunate that so many patients who are in great need of magnesium are not receiving it from their doctors.

Anaemia

The most common nutritional deficiency disease in the Western world is anaemia – a condition in which the red blood cells are not able to absorb enough oxygen. Most of us are familiar with the effects of anaemia: fatigue, shortness of breath and a pounding heart when you try to climb stairs. But severe anaemia can also cause water retention.

Normally assumed to be due to iron deficiency, most anaemia is treated with iron supplements and an iron-rich diet of red meat, liver and green vegetables. Vegetarians, who eat no meat, need to be aware that iron in plant foods is not well absorbed unless the meal also contains plenty of vitamin C.

Anaemia can cause water retention in two ways. First, severe anaemia seems to encourage the kidneys to retain sodium. As we know, this leads to water retention. Second, severe anaemia which goes on for too long can damage the heart. The heart works harder and harder as it tries to get the blood as fast as possible to the lungs for more oxygen. Eventually it starts to fail and has difficulty pumping blood at all. Reduced pumping means low fluid pressure in the kidneys and severe water retention.

While iron deficiency anaemia is the most common type, other deficiencies can also cause anaemia:

folic acid
vitamin B_2
vitamin B_6
vitamin B_{12}
vitamin C
vitamin E
copper
zinc
protein

A lack of any these nutrients causes anaemia by impairing the formation of healthy red blood cells.

Macrocytic anaemia, in which there are too few red blood cells and the cells become abnormally large and malformed, is caused by deficiencies of vitamin B_{12} and folic acid.

Pernicious anaemia, caused by a failure to absorb vitamin B_{12}, is a type of macrocytic anaemia.

Sickle cell anaemia is due to abnormal haemoglobin (the oxygen-carrying part of the red blood cell), which results in distorted and fragile red blood cells. Plasma levels of vitamin B_6 can be abnormally low in people who have this disease. Research reported in the *American Journal of Clinical Nutrition* in 1984 suggests that people with sickle cell anaemia can greatly benefit from supplementation with 100 mg of vitamin B_6 per day. The supplements can increase both the number of red blood cells and the haemoglobin levels. This suggests that sickle cell patients have much higher vitamin B_6 needs than the rest of the population.

Women taking the contraceptive pill also need to be careful not to develop vitamin B_6-related anaemia.

Essential polyunsaturated oils

Both magnesium and vitamin B_6 are among the nutrients which help to turn the essential polyunsaturated oils in your diet into prostaglandins. As we saw in Chapter 7, prostaglandins are hormone-like substances which help to control your body fluid levels, blood pressure and many other functions. They only act 'locally', which means that they may cause water retention in one of your joints, for example, while leaving the rest of your body unaffected. Prostaglandins are produced within the cell membrane – the delicate protective sheath which surrounds each cell. Apart from magnesium and vitamin B_6, the other important nutrients needed to make prostaglandins are zinc, biotin, selenium, iron and vitamins B_3, C and E.

Balancing your prostaglandins

Some prostaglandins are made from a fatty acid known as arachidonic acid, found in animal products: the fatty part of meat, dairy products and eggs. Prostaglandins derived from arachidonic acid promote water retention by increasing the leakiness of your blood capillaries and encouraging inflammation such as skin rashes or pain and swelling in joints. Other types of prostaglandins control the inflammatory ones by helping to prevent your cell membranes from releasing too much arachidonic acid.

The best way to control arachidonic acid is to avoid consuming animal products. Regularly consuming oily fish or cod liver oil also helps. Although your body does need small amounts of arachidonic acid, it can satisfy these needs by making it from other fats and oils.

The value of oily fish

Correcting your vitamin and mineral deficiencies will in time bring about the enzyme repairs needed to keep your prostaglandins in the right balance. In the meantime, a portion of so-called 'oily fish' such as salmon, sardines, pilchards, herrings or mackerel every few days will help you make more beneficial anti-inflammatory, anti-fluid-retention prostaglandins. (These fish are recommended as part of the Waterfall Diet.) In fact, this could be the reason why some women with premenstrual water retention derive so much benefit from eating a diet rich in these fish. The fish oils are acting as a medicine, altering the women's body chemistry.

Dr William Rea, Professor of Environmental Medicine at the University of Surrey in England, points out that excessive amounts of inflammatory prostaglandins are found in people suffering from a wide variety of chronic illnesses, including asthma and arthritis as well as premenstrual syndrome. Nutritional experts who specialise in this field are blaming this on deficiencies of the vitamins and minerals which help to make the anti-inflammatory prostaglandins.

HOW OILS ARE BROKEN DOWN TO PROSTAGLANDINS

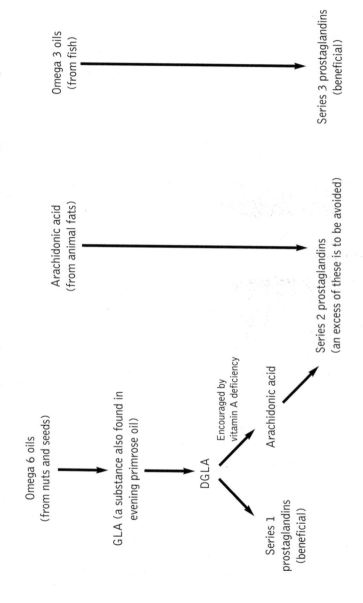

Omega 6 oils
(from nuts and seeds)

GLA (a substance also found in
evening primrose oil)

DGLA

Encouraged by
vitamin A deficiency

Arachidonic acid

Series 1
prostaglandins
(beneficial)

Series 2 prostaglandins
(an excess of these is to be avoided)

Arachidonic acid
(from animal fats)

Omega 3 oils
(from fish)

Series 3 prostaglandins
(beneficial)

To supplement or not?

Most fish oil supplements are not very strong and contain only a fraction of the active nutrient (known as EPA) found in oily fish themselves. The best brands of fish oil are those produced to 'pharmaceutical grade'.

Supplements of evening primrose oil, blackcurrant seed oil and borage oil can also be used to alleviate premenstrual syndrome and inflammation. The active ingredient in these supplements is known as GLA. But GLA can be turned either into anti-inflammatory prostaglandins or into much less desirable arachidonic acid. Professor Rea warns that a vitamin A deficiency may encourage the latter. Perhaps it would be a good idea for vitamin manufacturers to put some vitamin A (with zinc, which is often deficient and helps the body to use this vitamin) in their evening primrose oil products. Research using evening primrose oil to treat eczema, arthritis and PMS might then produce more consistently successful results in clinical trials.

One reason why so many arthritis sufferers seem to benefit from taking cod liver oil supplements is that cod liver oil does not just contain beneficial fish oils but is also a rich source of vitamin A. If you do take cod liver oil, try to find a purified brand, as some brands of fish oil can contain pollutants.

Flavonoids

As explained in Chapter 7, if the walls of your blood capillaries are weakened, they can leak protein-rich fluid into your tissue spaces. This weakness is known as capillary fragility. As long ago as the 1930s it was discovered that one particular type of nutritional deficiency was especially likely to cause capillary fragility. The nutrients concerned are known as flavonoids (or sometimes by the more old-fashioned term 'bioflavonoids'). They are powerful antioxidants found in fruit and vegetables, and are responsible for some of their colours such as the red or blue of grape and berry skins. Apart from their antioxidant properties, flavonoids are known for their ability to prevent and treat bruising, varicose veins, bleeding gums and nosebleeds. They may also be useful to treat some types of heavy menstrual bleeding. A third beneficial effect of the flavonoids quercetin, rutin, curcumin, silymarin and green tea polyphenols is their reputed anti-inflammatory effect, which works in a similar way to aspirin.

It is often said that flavonoids work by 'strengthening' the capillaries and that this is why they improve the circulation, eyesight and intellect. It implies that the foods containing them need only be consumed – like a kind of medicine – if you have circulatory problems. In fact flavonoids are not a treatment but an essential part of your diet. If you don't get enough of them from fruit and vegetables, your capillaries will weaken and become fragile.

Lemons (outer skin and white pith) and the central white core of all citrus fruit are a rich source of flavonoids. The white pith of green peppers is also good, as is the skin of colourful berries and grapes. Some herbs such as ginkgo biloba are taken partly for the action of their flavonoids.

Some common flavonoids

Name	Found in	Benefits
Anthocyanidins	Blue pigment (may appear red under acidic conditions) found in berry skins, especially bilberries	Beneficial effects on eyesight and circulation. Some antibacterial action.
Hesperidin	Citrus pith	Prevents capillary fragility. Anti-allergic: helps to minimise the effects of histamine.
Myricetin	Ginkgo biloba	Helps to prevent free radical damage to nerve cells.
Nobiletin	Citrus fruits	Has anti-inflammatory action and aids detoxification.

Table continued ▶

Some common flavonoids

Name	Found in	Benefits
Proanthocyanidins (also known as pycnogenols)	Pine bark, tea, peanut skins, cranberries, grape seeds and skins	Their antioxidant potency (particularly the varieties found in grape seeds) is reputedly twenty times greater than that of vitamin E.
Quercetin	Apple peel, onions, tea, ginkgo biloba and cabbage. Can also be synthesised by intestinal bacteria from rutin (*see below*)	Related to the anti-allergic drug disodium chromoglycate, quercetin may help allergy-related problems such as hay fever, asthma and eczema. It also decreases the synthesis of inflammatory prostaglandins. Research has shown that it helps prevent eye cataracts which can lead to blindness.
Rutin	Buckwheat and buckwheat tea	Helps in the treatment of high blood pressure, bruising and haemorrhages under the skin, including redness due to radiation. Has been used in the treatment of varicose veins.
Silybin	The herb milk thistle and its extract silymarin	Silymarin is a well-researched liver protective and regenerative substance which also protects cell membranes against damage by toxins.

Flavonoids and Type II water retention

Dr John Casley-Smith has carried out extensive research with the flavonoids rutin and quercetin and the related substance coumarin. He has found that not only can leaky capillaries repair themselves when these substances are consumed, but the number of white blood cells known as macrophages increases in areas where Type II water retention has developed. The macrophages produce enzymes which split the excess proteins in the tissue spaces into fragments that can finally be reabsorbed by the capillaries. Once the excess protein has been removed, the inflammation ceases and the excess fluid drains away into the blood or lymph.

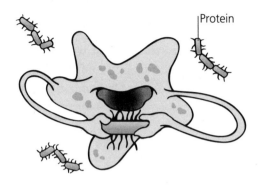

Protein

A macrophage

Natural medicine practitioners have always treated inflammatory conditions, such as arthritis and skin rashes, with 'cleansing'
diets of fruit and vegetables and their juices. Large amounts of
flavonoids can be consumed in such diets and may well account
for many success stories. Having endured scorn for decades from
other areas of the medical profession, natural medicine practitioners are delighted that so much modern research is confirming
the value of their nutritional treatments.

As we saw in Chapter 7, capillary walls can also be weakened
by a vitamin C deficiency, and lymphology experts have found
that vitamin C supplements can also help to reduce Type II water
retention.

Ginkgo biloba as a treatment for chronic water retention

The herb ginkgo biloba, a rich source of flavonoids, has been sub-
jected to numerous clinical trials to improve the circulation,
especially in the brain of elderly people. French kidney specialist
Dr G. Lagrue of the Henri Mondor Hospital in Créteil, France,
successfully used it on fifteen women who had tested positive for
leaky capillaries and Type II water retention. The most severely
affected women lost 4–10 lb of fluid, and the rest had good to

excellent results. This trial was published in the prestigious French medical journal *La Presse Médicale* in 1986.

For the cause of water retention in women, Dr Lagrue proposes a theory which is interesting to compare with Dr Abrahams' theory on PMS (*see p.116*). While Dr Abrahams proposes vitamin B_6 deficiency as the reason why the kidneys retain sodium and water, Dr Lagrue blames a deficiency of the female hormone progesterone. At the same time, says Dr Lagrue, the woman's capillaries are too leaky. This makes protein pass into her tissue spaces, where it attracts water. As her blood becomes more dehydrated, her body releases hormones to make her retain sodium and excrete less water. He proposes a two-fold treatment: giving progesterone artificially and treating the leaky capillaries with flavonoids.

Although Dr Lagrue does not suggest this treatment specifically for premenstrual water retention, there is no reason why it would not work. Dr Lagrue substitutes flavonoids for Dr Abrahams' vitamin B_6 treatment, but flavonoids and B vitamins often seem to have a similar therapeutic effect on leaky blood vessels. In fact, Dr Casley-Smith points out that flavonoids may be able to substitute for B vitamins in this respect.

Dr Abrahams says that a deficiency of progesterone is often caused by high oestrogen levels in the body and that a good way to raise progesterone levels is to boost the liver enzymes which break down excessive oestrogen. The way to do this is to ensure the liver gets enough magnesium and B vitamins. These nutrients are essential to make liver enzymes which process oestrogen. Consuming a magnesium-rich daily diet of wholegrains, sesame seeds and steamed or stir-fried green vegetables (as in the Waterfall Diet) together, if necessary, with magnesium supplements, would be a very sensible precaution if you are a PMS sufferer. Oestrogen levels can also rise if your diet is deficient in iodine and in vegetables from the Brassica family (broccoli, cauliflower, Brussels sprouts and cabbage).

Coumarin

Coumarin, a substance related to flavonoids, gives hay its characteristic sweet smell and is found in clover flowers, red wine, orange pith, red peppers, parsley, celery, horse chestnuts and many other foods and herbs. It is also effective against Type II water retention when applied as a cream, for instance to an arthritic joint. Although it appears to be little used outside Germany and Switzerland, your doctor should be able to prescribe it for you if your pharmacist is prepared to order it from international suppliers (*see Useful Addresses on p.276*).

Quercetin and rutin may also have an anti-allergy effect. As we know, allergic reactions involve the release of histamine, which increases the leakiness of capillaries. Coumarin and several flavonoids have anti-histamine effects. So, apart from water retention, if your arthritis, eczema, migraine or other health problems are caused by allergy, you may want to eat more flavonoid-rich foods (*see the table on p.125*) or perhaps use a juice extractor to turn them into drinks. This makes it easy to consume much larger quantities.

Some common foods and herbs which contain coumarin

alfalfa
angelica
aniseed
asafoetida
bitter lettuce (leaf and sap)
boldo
cayenne (chilli pepper)
celery
chamomile flowers
fenugreek seeds

horse-chestnut extract
horseradish root
king's clover flowers
liquorice root
meadowsweet
nettle
parsley
red clover flowers
Siberian ginseng
wild lettuce
woodruff

Coumarin is better absorbed through the skin than by mouth. Make yourself the following special remedies:

Coumarin bath recipe
Clover can be found growing wherever there is grass: meadows, heaths, roadsides and so on. Pick a large bag of clover flowers and allow the flowers to dry in the sun. Coumarin levels in clover flowers rise after wilting and drying. Tie up a handful of the flowers in a piece of muslin and soak this in your bath water before having a bath.

Coumarin tea
Pour some boiling water on to a few dried clover flowers and drink as a tea. Flavour with other ingredients, too, if you wish, such as chamomile, which also contains coumarin.

Coumarin – a treatment for lymphoedema
One of the biggest challenges to lymphologists is a severe type of water retention known as lymphoedema, which occurs when the lymphatic system becomes obstructed. A major cause of

lymphoedema is cancer treatments such as radiotherapy or surgery. Surgical removal of the lymph nodes in the armpit or groin can make an arm or leg swell up to twice its normal diameter. Dr Casley-Smith uses pharmaceutical coumarin to treat these cases, but most doctors advise only compression bandages, raising the affected limb, exercise and perhaps massage.

In one coumarin trial, one group of mastectomy patients who had had their under-arm lymph nodes removed were given compression bandages and advised to exercise their arms and keep them raised as much as possible, while a second group was also given daily doses of coumarin. The patients' arm circumference was then measured at regular intervals. In the first group, average arm circumference steadily increased as time went by, while in the second group there was a slow but steady reduction amounting to 3.3 mm every 10 months. The second group also suffered less from bursting pains, cramps, tension and secondary acute inflammation.

In the UK, if you suffer from lymphoedema, you should be able to get coumarin on prescription. The best products are Lympedim® and Lympaction®, sourced from India and Australia respectively. You can also obtain coumarin in the USA if you have a doctor's prescription. Lympaction does not require a doctor's prescription. (*See Useful Addresses on p.276.*)

Selenium helps lymphoedema caused by radiotherapy
A fairly recent treatment for lymphoedema is the trace element selenium. In 2003, a clinical trial carried out at the Münster University Hospital in Germany revealed that selenium supplements can help to reduce lymphoedema caused by radiotherapy. In this trial the supplements resulted in a 60 per cent reduction in arm circumference after only four to six weeks.

Safety

Don't worry – even when the individual flavonoids are extracted and sold as dietary supplements, they have not been found to cause any toxicity problems in clinical trials. Quercetin and rutin are not harmful.

Coumarin, too, is generally safe, although difficult to obtain in concentrated form. It has sometimes mistakenly been stigmatised as a human liver toxin, but this is not quite accurate. It is a liver toxin for certain species of animals, but humans, and animals with a similar metabolism to humans, are only rarely harmed by it. Occasional (one in 300–400) users of medically prescribed pharmaceutical coumarin develop liver inflammation after some months of use, so these products should be taken under medical supervision. Doctors who are experienced in prescribing pharmaceutical coumarin advise their patients to come back if they feel 'really unwell'. They are then given liver function tests and coumarin is stopped if the tests show there is a problem. The liver then returns to normal.

Coumarin is not the same substance as the blood-thinning drug warfarin, although confusion often arises between the two. While sometimes also referred to as coumarin, warfarin in fact consists of dicoumarin – a derivative of coumarin.

Selenium is potentially toxic in high doses, but doses of up to 200 micrograms a day are considered safe.

Nutritional deficiencies

How common are they?

We have referred a great deal to 'nutritional deficiencies' as causes of leaky capillaries and other problems leading to water retention. But most people who eat an average diet never really think about whether their body is getting enough vitamins and minerals, essential polyunsaturated oils and so on, and most have never even heard of flavonoids.

Orthodox nutritionists and doctors maintain that nutritional deficiencies are very rare in the western world, although they acknowledge that certain groups of people may be at risk: expectant mothers, dieters, the elderly, children and vegetarians.

However, clinical trials published in some of the world's most eminent medical and nutritional journals have found that certain very common 'incurable' health problems can disappear when consumption of a particular vitamin, mineral or other nutrient is increased. What does this mean? Certainly that some people have much higher needs for these nutrients than others. If those needs are not being met, is the person in question suffering from a nutritional deficiency?

In carrying out the research for my earlier book *The Nutritional Health Bible*, I came across hundreds of these trials published since the mid-1980s alone. Since few doctors now take much notice of clinical trials published in the 1950s and 1960s, I did not include these in the book, but in those days vitamin research was in its heyday as medical workers tried to find out whether any more so-called 'mystery' diseases like pellagra and beri-beri were really just nutritional deficiencies.

Now all this research has been largely forgotten, which is sad for the people who could benefit from the knowledge gained. A good example is schizophrenia. Dr Abram Hoffer was a practising psychiatrist during the heyday of nutritional medicine research. He was converted to the nutritional approach after the many successes he achieved with it, and is still active today, in Canada. He is quite sure that schizophrenia is a disease caused primarily by vitamin B_3 deficiency. He points out that there is no difference between the symptoms of schizophrenia and pellagra, the vitamin B_3 deficiency disease. They are so similar that in 1940s America after it was shown that vitamin B_3 could cure pellagra, psychiatric patients were given supplements of the vitamin. If they responded to it, they received a diagnosis of pellagra. If not they were labelled with schizophrenia. But some patients labelled with schizophrenia were subsequently given extra-large amounts of vitamin B_3 – up to 50 times the normal daily intake from food – and only then recovered.

What causes nutritional deficiencies?

There are still parts of the world where people suffer starvation and malnutrition. So how can we presume to talk about 'nutritional deficiencies' in the affluent West?

The problem here is that it is not usually a lack of food which leads to deficiency but ignorance about healthy eating. Many people have no idea of their body's nutritional needs. A recent survey I was involved in found that relatively few children nowadays are ever given a proper meal with fresh vegetables. In the UK at least, a whole generation of young people has grown up eating little other than chips, burgers, crisps and chocolate, with most of their knowledge of nutrition based on television advertisements for highly processed foods.

Healthy eating does not mean eating the occasional portion of spinach when you remember. As in the Waterfall Diet, it is about eating several portions of fresh fruit and vegetables every day, as well as making sure that most of your bread is wholemeal, and balancing the rest of your diet too. This really will minimise your risk of getting a diet-related illness.

But the story does not end here. What about the schizophrenia sufferers who did not become well until they were given vitamin B_3 supplements fifty times stronger than the normal intake? The children with asthma who can come off medication if they take fifty or a hundred times the normal intake of vitamin B_6 but not less? And the PMS sufferers who do not lose their symptoms unless they take strong B vitamin and magnesium supplements? There are many more examples in the medical literature. These people seem to have a greatly increased need for certain vitamins – far more than could be obtained from diet alone.

Is malabsorption the culprit?

There is still much that we do not know or understand about the human body. If some people can only lose their symptoms by taking nutritional supplements, it makes sense that there is something wrong with their ability to absorb nutrients.

Absorption takes place at several levels. The first involves your digestion. If you do not produce enough acid in your stomach (and it is said that 40 per cent of people over 60 do not), then the rest of your digestive processes may not be properly triggered. If you do not digest your food properly, it will not be broken down into small enough particles to nourish your body.

Food allergies, harmful bacterial or yeast overgrowth are some of the things that can mildly inflame your intestines and so impair food absorption. They cause symptoms such as:

bloating
discomfort after eating
excessive gas
irritable bowel syndrome

Once nutrients have been absorbed into your blood, they still have to be assimilated into the cells which use them. Many do not simply pass from your blood to your cells, but require special mechanisms. Virtually nothing is known about how factors like water retention, virus damage, chemical toxins and pollutants or lack of oxygen affect assimilation. We do know that your cells can be fooled by certain pollutants (for example, instead of calcium your nerve cells can absorb lead, which makes them malfunction). It is also known that water retention dilutes the material in your tissue spaces, which probably reduces assimilation.

Finally, people who have suffered severe vitamin B deficiency, such as former inmates of World War II Japanese prison camps, and those who had the B_3 deficiency disease pellagra in 1930s America, are known to have developed such abnormally high

needs for vitamin B₃ supplements that they must have had barely
any assimilation ability left at all.

How do you know if you have extra-large needs for certain nutrients?

If you eat a very good diet but still have some of the symptoms of
nutritional deficiency listed on pages 215–6, it is possible that you
might have extra-large needs. To find out for certain, you can have
'functional' tests carried out. These tests measure not the amount
of a nutrient in your blood but the enzymes in your body which
depend on that nutrient. Most functional tests are relatively new,
and although a few family doctors are using them you will probably need to have them done privately through a nutritional
therapist (*see Useful Addresses on p.276*).

In any event, reducing water retention with the Waterfall Diet
is sure to help improve the uptake of oxygen and nutrients by
your cells, which can only mean better health for your skin, hair,
eyes, bones, hormones, brain, nerves and arteries, and more
energy and vitality for you.

Heart disease can cause water retention

What most people refer to as 'heart disease' is actually coronary
heart disease (CHD), a disease of the coronary arteries which
supply your heart muscle with blood. Another type of heart disease is known as congestive heart failure (CHF), the main
symptom of which is severe water retention.

How does heart disease develop?
Cholesterol deposits on the coronary artery walls can eventually
reduce the blood supply, leaving your heart short of oxygen. If the
arteries become very narrow, angina pain occurs whenever you
exert yourself. Complete oxygen starvation, as when a small clot

---

lodges in the artery, is experienced as a heart attack (when part of the heart tissue dies) or cardiac arrest – the heart stops functioning completely.

After a heart attack, the tissue damage often leads to abnormalities in your heart's structure and reduced efficiency. As your heart struggles to keep up with its workload, it may in time start to fail; its pumping action may become unable to get blood around your body fast enough to keep all your organs supplied with enough oxygen and nutrients. This condition is known as congestive heart failure. The heart will often become enlarged as it attempts to work harder, and water retention can be a big problem.

People with congestive heart failure absorb less and less oxygen and develop fatigue, a chronic dry cough, shortness of breath and a bluish tinge to the lips.

Congestive heart failure can also develop without any previous damage to your heart, if your heart's workload becomes abnormally large for too long. Severe anaemia, for example, when the red blood cells are not able to absorb enough oxygen from the lungs, forces the heart to pump much harder as it attempts to get the blood around to the lungs again as quickly as possible. Other conditions which can damage the heart or increase its workload and so possibly lead to enlarged heart and CHF include:

alcohol abuse
severe vitamin B_1 deficiency
untreated high blood pressure
thyroid abnormalities
the lung diseases emphysema, asthma and chronic bronchitis
severe water retention
severe overweight

Standard medical treatments for CHF are restricted to treating the symptoms: diuretic drugs to reduce the water retention, other drugs to dilate your blood vessels, slow your heart rate and help it to pump, and advice to avoid excitement and exertion. Some doctors will also prescribe a low-salt diet. But research shows that a great deal more can be done for this life-threatening illness.

A combination of treatments

Natural treatments for CHF are used in addition to conventional treatments, and centre around the causes.

- Does the patient have a long-standing vitamin B_6 deficiency or food allergy which caused the original water retention?
- What about magnesium deficiency, associated with asthma and high blood pressure?
- Was he/she very deficient in flavonoids, and so developed leaky capillaries and inflammation in the lungs after breathing in fumes or smoke, possibly progressing to chronic bronchitis and emphysema?

If you or a relative are determined to do your very best to combat this illness, the Waterfall Diet will give you a very good start, since it is so rich in all the right nutrients. For the same reason it will help to reduce cholesterol levels and some people find that problems like angina and high blood pressure start to disappear.

Effective supplements

There is more good news. Several nutritional supplements have been found helpful against CHF, although they are not cures. One substance made by your body, known as coenzyme Q_{10}, is often deficient in patients with heart failure according to the medical journal *Clinical Investigations* (vol. 71 (supplement), pp.51–4,

1993). It also reported that heart failure patients with more coenzyme Q_{10} or vitamin E in their blood live longer.

Clinical trials, particularly in Italy, have now been carried out to see whether giving CHF patients 100 mg coenzyme Q_{10} per day could make a difference. The results have been reported in several medical journals: patients feel less tired, their ability to tolerate normal activity increases and they lose their breathing difficulties when resting.

Another nutritional supplement which has been found to be valuable in the treatment of CHF is the amino acid taurine. This nutrient regulates calcium and potassium in heart muscle cells and in nerve impulses in the heart. Since magnesium is also involved in potassium balance, taurine is sometimes combined with magnesium and sold as a supplement known as magnesium taurate.

CHAPTER 9

A swollen tummy:
Can it be caused by stress?

This chapter explains how stress can make you over-produce a hormone which encourages both water retention and the accumulation of fat around your middle.

Case report: Vivacious Valerie was in a state of emergency

Valerie worked as a teaching assistant for more than 30 years. Her weight had been steadily climbing since her forties. Now in her late sixties, she weighed 18 stone (252 lb). Her husband weighed 90 lb less than she did, although she ate less than him. Valerie rarely drank alcohol, ate no sugary foods or chocolate, as she was borderline diabetic, and walked up and down a steep hill most days to go shopping.

Valerie was the kind of lady who talked nineteen to the dozen. She was a darling, but everyone around her felt tired just trying to keep up with her excited chatter. It really was a little bit too much. While appearing to be quite jolly, her chatter and incessant entertaining stories about everyone and everything, were driven by a need to be the life and soul of the party – even when there was no party. This is stressful for anyone; Valerie barely paused to take breath while talking, and her pulse was permanently racing. She was on medication to control her blood pressure.

You would imagine that this endless stress would make Valerie thin rather than overweight, but this doesn't necessarily follow. Valerie's adrenal glands were pumping out stress hormones such as adrenaline and cortisol – hormones designed for dealing with emergency situations. But when you are in a more or less permanent state of emergency, they can have very profound effects on your body. Continually high levels of cortisol in particular cause weight gain, especially around the middle of your body. In fact, stress-related weight gain makes it possible to have a very big tummy while the rest of you remains thin.

How stress makes you fat

Cortisol is needed for most processes in the body. It helps to regulate blood pressure and kidney function, glucose levels, fat accumulation, protein synthesis and immunity. It also helps your thyroid gland to work more efficiently. In fact, if you make too much cortisol, or not enough, your thyroid hormones can be partially 'blocked'. In other words, it is possible to have normal levels of thyroid hormones in your blood, at the same time as having symptoms of thyroid deficiency or hypothyroidism. But your thyroid hormones govern your metabolism and energy production, so are very important if you want to avoid gaining weight.

As explained by biochemist Dr David Zava, Ph.D, director of ZRT Laboratory in Portland, Oregon, USA, what happens is that high cortisol levels, which occur when you are under stress, make your body's tissues develop a 'resistance' to your thyroid hormones. In other words your body stops responding to thyroid and behaves as if little or no thyroid is present. The same thing happens to other important hormones such as insulin, oestrogen and progesterone. When cortisol is high you have to make more insulin than usual in order to get energy from your blood sugar. It is also a very odd phenomenon that high cortisol levels can trigger a resistance to cortisol itself. In other words, the more cortisol you make, the more your body needs to make in order to get the desired results. No wonder chronic stress is such a drain on your strength and energy; none of your hormones are allowed to work properly. High cortisol levels also cause water retention and suppress your immune system, making you more vulnerable to colds and flu as well as cancers.

Finally, when you are perhaps approaching middle age, the deadly combination of high cortisol, high insulin and thyroid resistance will little by little make you begin to store fat rather than use it for energy. The type of fat which increases as a result of stress is your 'visceral' or internal body fat. This is not the layer of fat on the outside of your body, but the fat inside your body which surrounds your organs. It is very hard to lose internal fat.

Pear shape good, apple shape bad

In 2000, researchers at the University of California tested the stress levels of women with different waist measurements. They found that those with the most internal fat (those whose waist measurement was nearly as big as, or even bigger than their hips) appeared to be the most vulnerable to stress and had the highest cortisol levels.

If your internal fat continues to increase, there comes a point when it will start to get inflamed. We know this because large numbers of white blood cells known as macrophages are found in the internal fat of people with a big tummy. As we know, wherever there is inflammation there is usually also water retention.

Macrophages produce proteins which promote inflammation.

It is now believed that these proteins – known as cytokines – are partly responsible for some of the complications which have been linked with obesity, including heart disease and Type II diabetes. Excess amounts of internal fat seem to cause these problems rather than the fat on the outside of your body. In fact, researchers nowadays measure your waist-to-hip ratio in order to assess your risk of getting heart disease and diabetes. A body with a pear shape is good, but one with an apple shape is at risk.

Calculate your waist-to-hip ratio (WHR)

You will need a measuring tape and a calculator.

1. Gently breathe out and relax.
2. Without holding in your tummy, measure your waist circumference. You can use inches or centimetres. Do not pull the tape too tight.
3. Measure your hip circumference around the fullest part of your bottom.
4. Using your calculator, divide the waist measurement by the hip measurement. For example, if your waist is 36 inches and your hips are 42 inches, then divide 36 by 42. The answer is 0.85, which is your waist-to-hip ratio.

Use the chart below to assess your health risks.

Waist-to-hip ratio chart

Health risk based on WHR	Male	Female
Low risk	0.95 or less	0.80 or less
Moderate risk	0.96 to 1.0	0.81 to 0.85
High risk	1.0 or higher	0.85 or higher

Reducing stress

To get rid of excess internal fat and its inflammation and water retention, you first have to do everything you can to reduce stress. Assess your life. Is your job, relationship or home causing you a lot of stress? If you've been thinking of making a change, maybe start to think about it more seriously.

Do you get stressed for no reason? Are you nervous and anxious or highly excitable? Are you perhaps an aggressive, driven ('Type A') kind of person? Do you drive yourself too much without getting enough rest and relaxation? Or are you like Valerie – feeling duty-bound to be always laughing, always jolly, always the life and soul of the party? If you feel exhausted at the end of every day then it's likely you are over-stressed.

There are many natural therapies to help people reduce stress in their lives. Psychotherapy and hypnotherapy are obvious choices if you feel you can't control stress on your own. Homoeopathy, acupuncture and shiatsu can help to rebalance your nervous system and make you feel calmer and sleep better. Meditation can guide you to a different way of looking at your life. Some people find that exercise is a good stress release. But getting sufficient sleep and relaxation is probably the most important way of all to reduce stress and cortisol levels.

Some foods such as sugar and stimulants can create stress in your body if eaten to excess. The Waterfall Diet helps you as it avoids these foods completely for a while to give your body a rest from them.

Reducing inflammation

Cortisol is your body's natural anti-inflammatory hormone. It is not just released when you are under mental or physical stress, but also when you suffer from infections, allergic reactions or food intolerances. Many people have mild ongoing inflammation in their intestines as a result of food intolerances or irritation from intestinal bacteria. This inflammation alone can cause bloating and a swollen tummy due to water retention in the inflamed area. Cortisol is released in an attempt to keep the inflammation under control but high levels of cortisol can also increase amounts of internal fat. So to keep down the cortisol it's important to do everything you can to reduce inflammation.

The Waterfall Diet aims to help you discover your food intolerances, if any, and avoid any offending foods. It is low in sugar – which encourages the growth of irritating intestinal yeasts and bacteria – and rich in foods such as garlic, spices and olive oil, which help to control them. Oily fish such as salmon and sardines, as well as fish oil supplements, have a strong anti-inflammatory effect. My book *Treat Yourself with Nutritional Therapy* covers the subject of intestinal health in more detail.

A herbal product which may help to reduce cortisol and the effects of stress is Siberian ginseng. This is a different plant from the more commonly available Panax (red) or Korean ginseng.

Foods which can help to reduce internal fat

An interesting research study published in the December 2007 issue of the *Fertility and Sterility* journal tested soy on fifteen postmenopausal women to see if it could help reduce their internal fat. The women's measurements were taken and they were then given a daily soya milkshake plus concentrated soy extracts for three months. At the end of this period their measurements were taken again and compared with those of women who had received a dummy treatment. The result was quite unexpected. The women on the soy programme had a 14.7 square centimetre reduction in their visceral fat, whereas the women on the dummy treatment had a 22.9 square centimetre increase. This is very encouraging research indeed, as women are very prone to gaining internal body fat after the menopause.

Another food which shows promise is liquorice root. Liquorice contains the flavonoid glabridin, which has been shown to have an anti-inflammatory effect and to decrease internal fat. It works by reducing the rate of fat synthesis while increasing the activity of the enzymes which break down fat tissue.

In a carefully conducted double-blind trial in Japan, reported in the *Journal of Health Science* in 2006, 103 overweight people were supplemented with liquorice extract for 12 weeks. Compared with the group of people on the dummy treatment, they showed a significant reduction in body fat and body mass index (BMI). This success was repeated in another, subsequent, clinical trial carried out for eight weeks. The group treated with liquorice extract not only showed a reduction in overall fat, but specifically internal fat.

If you want to buy a liquorice product or supplement but have a tendency to high blood pressure, make sure you get one which has been 'deglycyrrhizined'. Glycyrrhizin, a component of liquorice, can raise the blood pressure if liquorice is consumed regularly. Deglycyrrhizined liquorice supplements have had the glycyrrhizin removed.

The black confectionery product sold as liquorice does not necessarily contain any liquorice. Some brands are just flavoured with aniseed.

Reasons for women to keep stress at bay

The menopause

When levels are high of the stress hormone cortisol, the brain is less sensitive to several hormones, including oestrogen. According to US hormone expert Dr John Lee, that's why menopausal women get hot flushes when they are in a mildly stressful situation. Even just a slightly anxious thought such as 'Did I remember to lock the back door?' can set off a hot flush. That's because cortisol is released, causing a temporary oestrogen 'deficiency'. It's not a real oestrogen deficiency, because even after the ovaries stop producing oestrogen most women still have plenty – sometimes too much – of this hormone in their system. We know this because after the menopause, conditions such as fibroids and breast cancer, which are caused by high oestrogen levels, are common. After the menopause it is another female hormone, progesterone, which declines much more steeply than oestrogen.

If you suffer from menopausal hot flushes I recommend that you try to balance your hormones by following the Waterfall Diet and the advice in the rest of this chapter. You may also benefit from natural herbal products such as agnus castus, black cohosh, dong quai, motherwort and sage to help control your hot flushes. Unlike artificial hormone replacement therapy (HRT), these herbs are not likely to cause water retention.

Another effect of too much stress on menopausal women is bone loss and an increased risk of osteoporosis, the brittle bone disease. Cortisol inhibits your ability to make and repair bone, speeds up bone and calcium loss and decreases your absorption of minerals from your diet.

Premenstrual swollen tummy

In Chapter 8 we briefly mentioned how premenstrual syndrome – a common cause of tummy swelling, water retention and bloating – can be caused by deficiencies of vitamin B_6 and magnesium, and also by too much oestrogen. Oestrogen can remain high if your diet lacks the nutrients which your liver needs to break it down. If oestrogen is not broken down sufficiently, your body can become overloaded with oestrogen and can also develop a corresponding lack of progesterone. Dr John Lee refers to this high oestrogen/low progesterone state as 'oestrogen dominance'. Not only does oestrogen dominance cause water retention and other premenstrual symptoms, it is also responsible for a host of female problems such as breast lumps, mood swings, excessive bleeding, endometriosis, fibroids, infertility and ovarian cysts. Women with too much oestrogen are also prone to put on fat more easily and find it hard to lose weight.

Other dietary imbalances can raise a woman's natural oestrogen levels. A low-fibre diet allows oestrogens found in bile (a liquid released by your gall bladder into your intestines) to be reabsorbed through a woman's intestines back into her blood instead of being excreted in her stools. High levels of fat in her diet also tend to alter hormone balance, and body fat itself makes substantial amounts of oestrogen.

Many environmental pollutants in the air, food and water, including pesticides, plastics and PCBs are chemically so similar to oestrogen that they are known as 'oestrogen mimics'. Once these chemicals get into the body they are hard to excrete and tend to accumulate in the body fat. They have an uncanny ability to masquerade as natural oestrogen and are taken up by the oestrogen receptor sites in the body, where they interfere with natural body processes. Other potential sources of oestrogen mimics include drinks sold in plastic bottles and tap water.

The Waterfall Diet to the rescue

One of the most important foods a woman can eat to help keep her hormones balanced is soy in the form of soya milk, soya yoghurt and tofu. The Waterfall Diet includes soy and other foods that help balance your hormones, break down excess oestrogen and clear it out of your body as quickly as possible.

CHAPTER 10

Swollen legs and ankles

This chapter looks at the causes of this very common problem and the research into herbs and foods that can help it, and gives a daily routine that you can use to help relieve it. There is also a section on swollen legs in pregnancy and advice on how to prevent pre-eclampsia, a dangerous condition which can occur in pregnancy and may be caused by water retention.

Case report: Dorothy – a case of swollen legs

Dorothy's legs and ankles seemed to be getting more and more swollen as she got older. Working in a shop, she was on her feet all day, which made the problem worse. She never got the chance to put her feet up. Eventually the problem got so bad that, especially in warm weather, her feet would no longer fit into her shoes and she had to buy a larger size. Ugly varicose veins which felt quite sore and painful were beginning to show on her legs, and some of the skin was very red and would bleed easily.

Dorothy's doctor didn't have much to suggest except for support stockings and 'putting her feet up'. 'Varicose veins usually get worse over time,' he said. 'If they get too bad you can have surgery to remove them if necessary.' Dorothy decided to try the Waterfall Diet and within six days she was saying 'I haven't seen my ankles this small in a long time'.

Swollen legs

Swollen legs are a common problem, especially in older or pregnant women. Various medical terms are used to describe swollen legs and ankles, including 'chronic venous insufficiency' and 'idiopathic cyclic oedema'.

Chronic venous insufficiency

Like all the veins in your body, those in your legs have to return blood to your heart. But this is more difficult in your legs, as the blood needs to flow upwards against gravity. When you are actively walking around, your calf muscles and the muscles in your feet contract with each step, massaging your veins and pushing your blood upwards. One-way valves in your veins help to keep the blood flowing upwards. Chronic venous insufficiency (CVI) occurs when these valves become damaged. When the valves are not working, the blood can drop back down again instead of continuing to travel upwards. As blood pools in your veins, the extra pressure forces capillaries to leak fluid into the tissue spaces of your lower legs, ankles and feet, making them swollen. Sometimes the pressure makes the veins themselves swell and bulge through the skin. This is a painful and unsightly condition known as varicose veins.

If the pressure and swelling continue to increase, the skin of the legs can start to leak tiny drops of plasma, which is the pale yellow fluid component of blood. Sometimes the capillaries burst under the high pressure, releasing red blood cells under the skin, which discolour it. The skin in these areas is easily broken, and prone to developing leg ulcers. People with chronic venous insufficiency find that their legs ache and feel tired or heavy, especially after long periods of standing.

'Thread' veins (small, discoloured veins visible under the skin) can be caused by constipation. Straining to have a bowel movement closes the veins in your legs, and the resulting pressure may restrict the flow of blood in your large veins and force too much blood to go through small, superficial veins instead.

Risk factors for developing venous insufficiency:

overweight
constipation
pregnancy
not enough exercise
a blockage such as a blood clot in an important vein
vein walls are too weak or slack
Type II water retention

Idiopathic cyclic oedema (ICO)

This is a condition in which the legs swell due to Type II water retention caused by leaky, fragile capillaries.

Conventional treatments for swollen legs

The conventional treatments for swollen legs and ankles are compression therapy (wearing compression stockings) and keeping the legs raised. Surgery may be recommended to remove varicose veins, but several non-surgical options are also available, including:

- Sclerotherapy: an injection of chemical solution into the vein, which closes it off, forcing other (hopefully stronger) veins to take over the blood flow.
- Microwaves: delivered by a fine tube inserted into the veins. This treatment causes the affected veins to collapse and shrink.

- Laser treatments: These heat up the affected veins, causing them to collapse and shrink.

None of these treatments correct the causes of chronic venous insufficiency such as Type II water retention and slack or flaccid veins.

Natural treatments for swollen legs

Some very interesting research studies have recently been conducted in countries with a strong tradition of natural medicine, including Germany, Italy, Mexico and Brazil. These studies may offer a much more lasting solution to the problem of swollen legs and ankles.

In 2008, a study carried out at the São José Medical School in Brazil was reported in the journal *Phlebology*. Fifteen women aged 22–49 with swollen legs, who had been diagnosed with ICO, were asked to record their body weight every morning and evening. The size of their legs was also measured. The women were given a medicine known as aminaphtone, which is derived from the vitamin-like compound PABA. Aminaphtone is used to treat excessively leaky capillaries. After five days, 70 per cent of the patients were found to have a significant reduction in the swelling.

Aminaphtone is not available over the counter, and there is no evidence that PABA supplements can do the job. But there may be an even more effective natural treatment. In 2007, the journal *International Angiology* reported the results of a study carried out at a hospital in Jalisco, Mexico. In this study, 124 patients with CVI were given a treatment consisting of a combination of the herb butcher's broom, the flavonoid hesperidin, and vitamin C supplements. After two weeks, symptoms such as pain, heaviness, cramps and water retention began to decrease, and by eight weeks they had disappeared completely. The patients' capillaries were evaluated and were found to be significantly less fragile. Butcher's broom (also known as *Ruscus aculeatus*) is a vein tonic; it helps to

---

Daily routine for swollen legs and ankles

- Before rising in the morning, lie on your back with your legs in the air, stretched as high as you can, and do 'cycling movements' with your legs. (Support your hips with your hands to help keep your balance.) Do this for a full minute if you can. It helps to get the circulation going in your legs, and empties the lymph nodes in your groin area.
- Next, with your legs still in the air, spend a further one to two minutes rotating and wiggling your ankles. This will help the lymph to flow through the nodes which you have just emptied.
- Finally, give your legs a gentle massage with cooling witch hazel gel or cream. During the course of the day, try to sit down a few times with your feet up and give your legs another massage. Walking is very helpful for swollen legs, so try to do as much as you can.

The Waterfall Diet on its own has helped many people with swollen legs and ankles, but to speed things up you may also want to add some of the herbs listed in this chapter. Horse chestnut, ginkgo biloba and butcher's broom are especially helpful. Just follow the directions on the product's packaging.

---

contract and strengthen the walls of veins so that they become less flaccid. Hesperidin (a flavonoid found in the white pithy part of orange peel) and vitamin C reduce capillary fragility and leakiness. This prevents excessive amounts of fluid from entering the tissue spaces and allows the lymphatic system the opportunity to drain away any existing excess fluid.

Another herb which has a beneficial effect on vein strength is an extract from horse chestnut seeds. A number of successful research studies have been carried out using this herb. In 2002, the journal *International Angiology* published an analysis of all these studies, carried out by the Institute of Medical Informatics, Biometry and Epidemiology, Ludwig-Maximilians University of Munich, Germany. Based on all the clinical trials and observations carried out to date, the researchers recommended horse chestnut as a safe, effective treatment for CVI. A 1996 article in the world-famous medical journal the *Lancet* reported that horse chestnut reduced water retention in patients with CVI almost as effectively as compression stockings. But unlike compression stockings, the herb corrected the cause of the problem.

In the same year, the *European Journal of Clinical Pharmacology* reported good results with a treatment based on flavonoids. This was a double-blind clinical trial carried out at Humboldt University in Berlin, Germany, in which patients with CVI drank buckwheat leaf tea for three months. At the end of the trial their legs had not got any worse and showed some improvement. In contrast the disease had progressed in those patients who were on the dummy treatment.

How to reduce swelling and varicose veins

- Wear support tights. Ankle socks may cut into your swollen legs but support tights that go up to the waist can help to control the swelling.
- Avoid too much standing still and put your feet up whenever possible. This helps to stop fluid collecting in your legs.
- Move your feet and ankles as often as you can when you do have to sit for extended periods. Rotate your ankles, stretch your legs and wiggle your toes. Get up and walk about occasionally.
- Don't cross your legs; this restricts your circulation.
- Wear comfortable shoes.

- Soak your feet in cool water.
- Drink plenty of water. This helps your kidneys and reduces water retention. When your body is well-hydrated it will not hold on to water.
- Get as much exercise as you can. Walking, swimming or dancing, for instance, will help to boost your circulation.
- Gently massage tired, aching legs with witch hazel cream.
- Exercise your calf muscles by standing up and lifting your heels off the floor so that you are standing on tip-toe. Do this quickly ten times, several times a day.
- In pregnancy, lie on your left side. During the later stages of pregnancy, lying on your back puts pressure on the vena cava vein. Lying on your left-hand side instead will help your blood to return to your heart instead of collecting in your legs.
- Heat can aggravate leg swelling and varicose veins. Instead of taking hot baths, try cool showers instead.
- Follow the Waterfall Diet. It will improve the integrity of your capillaries and it is low in salt and high in dietary fibre, which will help to prevent constipation.
- Regularly eat chillies or cayenne pepper, garlic, onion and ginger and drink pineapple juice. These foods are thought to help break down fibrin – a tough protein layer which can develop around the capillaries in swollen legs and further restricts the circulation.

An old folk remedy for varicose veins is apple cider vinegar. Apply a layer of vinegar-soaked bandage to the affected areas of your legs and leave for half an hour. At the same time, slowly drink a small glass of warm water containing two teaspoons of apple cider vinegar.

Water retention in pregnancy

Swelling of the legs and feet, and sometimes even the arms and hands, is common in late pregnancy. Few women go through the whole nine months without experiencing this to some extent. During pregnancy, levels increase of several hormones, such as cortisol, oestrogens, and progesterone. These hormonal changes alone can lead to some water retention, but there are other causes too. Swelling in the legs, ankles and feet is mostly caused by pressure from the uterus on a large vein in your pelvis. This vein is called the vena cava and carries blood from your lower body back to your heart. Pressure on this vein makes blood flow more slowly so that it pools in your legs and ankles. The extra pressure in your legs forces your capillaries to leak fluid into the tissue spaces of your legs. You may find that the swelling gets worse the more time you spend on your feet. Warm weather also tends to aggravate the problem.

During pregnancy, swollen feet, ankles, hands and arms are usually not serious and the swelling goes down after delivery. But if you develop any of the following symptoms:

> swelling or puffiness in your face or around your eyes
> severe swelling of your hands (more than just a tightness of your rings)
> sudden severe swelling of your feet and ankles
> swelling significantly worse in one leg than the other
> pain in your calves or thighs

you should seek medical attention straight away, as this could be a sign of a more serious condition known as pre-eclampsia.

Pre-eclampsia
Pre-eclampsia is a common complication of pregnancy. It consists of water retention, high blood pressure and protein in the urine.

It is not usually diagnosed until the second half of pregnancy. Pre-eclampsia is considered dangerous and can lead to convulsions and even to the baby's death. The cause is unknown, but as water retention raises the blood pressure it is likely that severe water retention could be a significant cause of pre-eclampsia.

High blood pressure is one of the leading causes of pregnancy-related death, accounting for 15 to 20 per cent of all maternal deaths in the developing as well as the developed world. It is also one of the leading causes of premature birth. If your doctor suspects that you have pre-eclampsia, he or she will check your urine for protein, using a urine dipstick. Pre-eclampsia will be diagnosed if you have both high blood pressure and protein in your urine. Protein in the urine is a sign that the blood pressure is too high for your kidneys. The capillaries in your kidneys are meant to drip fluid gently from your blood into tiny funnels which eventually channel the fluid to your bladder. Excessively high blood pressure forces protein as well as fluid through these capillaries and into your urine.

The medical treatment of pre-eclampsia includes bed rest, blood pressure-reducing drugs and preventing convulsions with injections of magnesium sulphate. Hospitalisation is sometimes recommended. Rest is important, as it improves the blood flow through the placenta. Delivery will be brought forward if convulsions, headaches or uncontrollable high blood pressure occur.

Research carried out at the University of Chile and at Laval University, Canada, suggests that one potential cause of pre-eclampsia is an inadequate intake of antioxidant nutrients. The researchers believe that supplementation with vitamins C and E may actually be helpful in preventing pre-eclampsia.

Inflammation

Inflammation is another potential contributor to water retention in pregnancy, especially if it affects the kidneys. Inflammatory illnesses such as lupus and nephritis are prone to flare up during pregnancy, probably due to increases in oestrogen. On the other hand, strangely enough, other inflammatory illnesses such as rheumatoid arthritis can partially disappear during pregnancy.

Cornsilk tea: A safe remedy for swollen legs in pregnancy

In his wonderful *Encyclopedia of Herbal Medicine*, Master Herbalist Thomas Bartram recommends drinking cornsilk tea for swollen ankles in pregnancy. Cornsilk is the silky strands found under the green outer sheath of a head of sweetcorn (maize). Historical records show that cornsilk extract was being used in the eighteenth century for its diuretic properties. It was also used for kidney, urinary tract and bladder infections, bed wetting problems, cystitis, liver or gall bladder complaints, arthritis and gout.

To make cornsilk tea, first collect the strands, leave them in a warm place for a few days until dry, then rub them together to break them up and place them in an airtight container. Put 1 oz (28 g) of dried cornsilk in a saucepan with 1 pint of water, bring to the boil, and keep boiling until reduced down to half a pint. Drink this tea twice a day.

You can also buy ready-made cornsilk products such as capsules or tinctures. To use these, simply follow the instructions on the packet.

Bartram also recommends that all pregnant women should drink raspberry leaf tea up to three times daily, with a few drops of liquid extract of Black Haw to prevent miscarriage. Raspberry leaf is easily available in health food stores and helps to tone the muscles of the uterus and aid a painless, easy delivery. It also promotes milk production.

Buckwheat leaf tea is also very helpful against water retention and swollen legs.

Swimming pool exercises

According to a 2005 research study carried out at Zurich University Hospital, Switzerland, exercising your legs under water may also help to reduce leg swelling in pregnancy. In this study, nine women with severely swollen legs took part in a 45-minute exercise session while immersed in water. The size of their legs was measured before and after the session. The average fluid loss was 8 fl oz (200ml), and the women also reported that their legs felt less swollen.

CHAPTER 11

Water retention remedies:
Foods, herbs and homeopathy

We have already mentioned many of the foods, nutrients and herbal remedies which can help combat water retention. This chapter, intended to be a useful reference section, goes into more detail on each of these items and also covers others which we have not yet discussed. Section II gives guidance on incorporating the foods into the Waterfall Diet.

Foods

Flavonoids

As we know, some foods are beneficial against water retention because they help to prevent your capillaries from getting too leaky. These are foods rich in vitamin-like compounds known as flavonoids.

The main flavonoids are the dark red, blue and purple pigments found in the skins of fruits such as black grapes, bilberries, blueberries, blackberries and black cherries. Citrus fruits such as oranges and tangerines are also rich in flavonoids of a different type. One of these flavonoids is named hesperidin, and is found in the white pithy part of citrus peel. Hesperidin has been tested as a treatment for swollen legs in clinical trials and is considered very effective, especially when used in combination with a herb known as butcher's broom (*see below under Herbs*).

Lemon zest (the outer, yellow skin of the lemon) is a rich source of quercetin, a flavonoid with a mildly anti-histamine and anti-inflammatory effect. Histamine is produced when inflammation or allergies are present. It causes capillary walls to stretch, which makes them leaky. Other foods rich in quercetin include onions, cabbage and the petals of red roses! You should eat plenty of quercetin-rich foods if your water retention is related to food allergies or intolerances (*see Chapter 2*). Quercetin also has benefits similar to those of coumarin (*see below*) and, like other flavonoids, it helps to repair fragile capillaries.

Although this remains to be researched, it's very likely that flavonoids benefit your kidneys too. The capillaries in your kidneys are extremely porous; their job is to drip fluid from your blood into tiny funnels which eventually channel the fluid to your bladder. Without sufficient flavonoids these capillaries could in theory become too porous, allowing protein and excess fluid to escape from your blood.

Wholegrains and brassicas

Other foods help to combat water retention by being rich in B vitamins, magnesium and other vitamins and minerals, which your body needs to maintain the intricate balance of hormones that governs how much you urinate. These foods include wholegrains such as oats, rye and brown rice, as well as leafy green vegetables. Other important vegetables are the cruciferous vegetables, sometimes known as brassicas. These include broccoli, cauliflower, cabbage and Brussels sprouts. They contain ingredients which help the liver to break down oestradiol. Remember that oestradiol is a potent form of oestrogen, high levels of which can cause a number of health problems for women, including water retention. It is really important that every woman's liver should be very efficient at breaking down unwanted oestradiol. High levels of oestradiol are not only linked with water retention but also with breast lumps, fibroids, ovarian cysts and endometriosis.

Soya products also help the liver to break down oestradiol (the most active form of oestrogen) though they act in a different way from the brassica vegetables. I don't recommend eating highly-processed soya products such as TVP (textured vegetable protein) or SPI (soya protein isolate), as there is a potential risk that these may cause hormonal imbalances. On the other hand, soya milk, soya yoghurt and tofu are absolutely fine when eaten as part of a balanced diet.

Protein

Eating enough protein is vital to maintain the right fluid balance. Protein attracts water, so, once digested and in your bloodstream, it can act like a useful magnet, drawing excess water out of your tissues and back into your blood. But don't make the mistake of thinking that the more protein you eat, the more water retention you will lose! A piece of meat or fish the size of the palm of your hand is more than enough protein if eaten twice a day. Many plant foods such as nuts, beans, lentils, soya products and rice are also good sources of protein.

Celery and parsley

These two foods are very useful in combating Type II water retention. If you remember, this is the type caused by inflammation, histamine or leaky capillaries. In Type II water retention too much protein escapes into your tissue spaces and then cannot get back again. Celery and parsley are rich in a substance known as coumarin. This encourages white blood cells known as macrophages to accumulate in the tissue spaces, where they 'digest' the excess protein, breaking it up into particles which are small enough to get back into the capillaries. Both celery and parsley are also natural diuretics – helping the kidneys to make urine.

Other foods rich in coumarin include alfalfa, asafoetida (a pungent Indian spice) and fenugreek seeds.

Caution

During pregnancy, it is fine to consume a little parsley in your food, but avoid using parsley or celery seeds for medicinal purposes.

Pineapples

Pineapples are said to aid the digestion. This is because the fruit, and more particularly the stems, are a good source of a natural enzyme known as bromelain. Bromelain is so effective at digesting food that it is isolated and put into capsules for use as a dietary supplement.

The protein-digesting properties of bromelain can also be used to help reduce swellings and Type II water retention. If you sprain your ankle, for instance, fluid and protein will leak from damaged capillaries and gather in the tissue spaces of your ankle, causing pain and swelling. When given by mouth as a supplement, bromelain can digest this protein. To see if it can help to speed up the healing of injuries, it has, with positive results, been given to athletes in clinical trials. Pain and swelling subside much more quickly than without the supplements. As the protein in the tissue spaces is broken down, the fluid which causes the swelling can return to the blood. And as the swelling subsides, so does the pain.

The stem of a pineapple extends upwards into the core of the fruit. This core is very tough and fibrous – not easy to eat. However it can be juiced along with the flesh of the pineapple, so pineapple juice is likely to be a good source of bromelain.

Radishes

Radishes and radish juice are very useful as a secondary treatment for water retention. They are a mild diuretic and also help to balance the thyroid gland and break down mucus. Mucus can build up in the body as a result of eating improperly digested foods. If your intestines are a little inflamed and allow particles of undigested wheat or dairy protein, for instance, to get into your blood, these proteins may be deposited in tissues and organs. These deposits stimulate the formation of mucus, which is intended to encapsulate them so that they can cause no harm. But if this mucus is allowed to build up, it can solidify and block the flow of oxygen and nutrients to cells, as well as the flow of lymph. Radish juice has mucus-dissolving properties and so can help to get things flowing again. By helping to balance the thyroid gland, radish juice is also beneficial to the metabolism in general. You can of course eat radishes, but you would not be physically able to eat enough of them to get a particularly therapeutic effect. One wineglass of radish juice is the equivalent of up to ten radishes.

In Traditional Chinese Medicine, radishes are thought to aid digestion and combat bloating. They can be eaten either raw or cooked. The long white radishes known as mooli or icicle radishes are especially good for juicing, but leave the juice to stand for 20 minutes before drinking it, to remove some of the pungency.

Other natural diuretics

Provided that you eat the right foods to combat Type II water retention, it will do no harm if you also eat foods that act as natural diuretics. Apart from parsley, celery and radishes, other foods with diuretic properties include cucumbers, watermelons, watercress, horseradish, lemons, cranberries, pomegranates, asparagus, carrots, celery seeds, fennel seeds and pumpkin seeds. As their diuretic effect is mild, you would need to consume large amounts to get the desired effect. Once again, it is easier to consume large amounts of these fruits and vegetables if you make them into juice.

Traditional Chinese Medicine

In Traditional Chinese Medicine, it is said that if you want to lose weight and stay slim, eat ginger, chives and garlic every day. These foods are 'yang tonics', which means that they help to balance the adrenal glands. Other yang tonics include shrimps, prawns, mussels, kidney and liver.

In Chinese medicine, cinnamon is highly regarded as a food which helps to drive excess water out of the body. Obesity is viewed as mostly a water retention problem. According to Chinese philosophy, the type of constitution that suffers from water retention tends to be either 'warm-damp' or 'cold-damp'. Certain foods (cinnamon, aduki beans, mung beans and cornsilk tea) can help to dry up excess water or (in the case of broad beans and tea made from dried broad bean pods) they can act like a sponge to soak it up. All pungent foods and spices such as ginger, chilli, cardamom, fennel seeds, pepper and cloves help to warm the body and contribute to driving off excess water, but must not be eaten to excess. If they burn your mouth or taste unpleasant, then you have put too much in your food.

Cornsilk tea is made by drying the silky strands found under the green outer sheath of a head of sweetcorn (maize) and boiling them in water before straining and drinking. (*See the recipe on page 158.*)

Herbs

Herbs for water retention fall into two categories: diuretics, and herbs which can combat Type II water retention by reducing inflammation, relieving lymphatic congestion or improving the blood circulation. Some herbs are also rich in coumarin, which as we know can help the body to break down proteins which have become trapped in the tissue spaces.

When taking herbal products, follow the instructions on the packet. Some herbs are available as tea products and others as pills or tinctures. If you buy tinctures, you can mix herbs together and drink them stirred into a glass of hot water. If you are planning to take more than four herbs on a daily basis it is best to consult a medical herbalist. Most of the herbs listed here are widely available because they are low in toxicity, but it is always best to be on the safe side, especially if you are pregnant, breastfeeding or perhaps planning pregnancy. Check the product labels carefully.

Diuretic herbs

Some common diuretic herbs include dandelion roots, bilberry leaves, lime flowers and juniper berries. These are gentle diuretics and so are suitable for individuals with Type II water retention, provided that they are consumed as part of the Waterfall Diet. Dandelion root is also sold as 'dandelion coffee' in the form of granules or dried root pieces to which you can add boiling water. Dandelion root is a really useful diuretic as it also helps to drain (or 'cleanse') the liver and gall bladder.

Anti-inflammatory herbs

These help to combat water retention caused by auto-immunity, allergies and other causes of inflammation or bloating such as intestinal bacteria. They include chamomile, fennel, turmeric (also used as a yellow spice in Asian cookery) and wild yam. Garlic has powerful anti-histamine properties; other herbs with anti-histamine properties include ginger, echinacea and peppermint.

Lymphatic herbs

Lymphatic herbs help to ease congestion in the lymphatic system and aid the flow of lymph. Traditionally, they include red clover, marigold petals, agnus castus, fenugreek seeds and burdock. Clivers is useful if the lymph glands are blocked and swollen.

Herbs rich in coumarin

These include angelica, boldo, chamomile flowers, horse chestnut extract, meadowsweet, nettle, red clover and Siberian ginseng.

Herbs for swollen legs and varicose veins

The following herbs help to support the veins and strengthen the valves which aid the flow of blood upwards from your legs and ankles: gotu kola, ginkgo biloba, horsetail, horse chestnut, butcher's broom, parsley and buckwheat (flowers and leaves). Buckwheat tea, for instance, is readily available to buy in health food stores, and, like most of these herbs, has been tested in clinical trials. In some countries, doctors prescribe both horse chestnut and butcher's broom for swollen legs and ankles.

If you have high blood pressure or if your doctor says that your swollen legs are due to a tired heart with poor pumping action, you may also want to consider taking hawthorn. This is a gentle herb which can help to reduce blood pressure and has many benefits for the heart.

Witch hazel gel or cream can be applied directly to soothe your legs, but do this very gently if you have varicose veins.

Homeopathy

Several homeopathic remedies can be potentially helpful in the treatment of water retention. When taking homeopathic remedies, the most suitable potencies are generally 6 or 30. Other potencies are best taken under the advice of a qualified homeopath. As long as you identify with the main characteristics described for a remedy, you can take it and it will do no harm. If you find it hard to choose between several remedies, you can mix them together and take up to four at a time. A homeopathic pharmacy can make up such a mixture for you. You should take your chosen remedy(ies) twice a day for at least two weeks.

Calc. carb.

Calc. carb. is best used by those with water retention in their legs, feet or ankles, who also feel tired and are exhausted by minor physical exertion.

Graphites

Graphites is best used by individuals with water retention who also put on weight very easily, and are prone to skin problems such as cracked skin behind the ears or on the fingertips.

Ledum

Ledum is useful to treat swellings caused by injuries or insect bites.

Lycopodium

Lycopodium is best used by individuals whose water retention is accompanied by digestive problems, bloating and gas, and often an extreme craving for sweets.

Nat. mur.

Nat. mur. is best used by those with water retention who have a tendency to hide their feelings and pretend that everything is fine even if it is not. There may also be a craving for salt and salty foods. Nat. mur. may also be useful for puffiness around the eye area, especially if this started as a result of an allergic reaction or exposure to sunlight.

Pulsatilla

Pulsatilla is best used by those with water retention, especially in the hands or feet, who also have a sensation of heaviness or weariness, and a tendency to feel sorry for themselves or get moody. The condition improves with fresh air and gentle exercise and deteriorates if the affected limb is allowed to hang down.

For help with finding suitable natural products, sign up for my e-mail newsletters at www.health-diets.net.

SECTION II

The Waterfall Diet

CHAPTER 12

Phase I of the Waterfall Diet: Goodbye to excess water weight

Now that you have identified some possible reasons why you might be retaining water, it is time for your treatment: the Waterfall Diet. This chapter summarises the instructions for the first part of the diet, which lasts for four weeks, and starts you off with a 7-day menu plan.

The Waterfall Diet is not a low-calorie diet. It is a medical diet which aims to treat up to seven different causes of water retention. Losing weight is a great bonus, but water retention can be responsible for quite a lot of other health problems, ranging from arthritis to premenstrual syndrome and even migraine. When you get rid of the excess water, you can often get rid of these problems too.

How does the diet work?

Almost all other diets aim to help you lose weight either by reducing calories (e.g. low-calorie and low-fat diets) or by influencing your metabolism (low-carb and GI diets). The Waterfall Diet works by taking away what might be making you retain water, finding out what foods are safe for you to eat and making you eat beneficial foods which help you to release excess water. It's as simple as that. The Waterfall Diet is not a low-calorie diet – in fact you are positively encouraged to eat normal portion sizes in order to get all the vitamins and minerals you need.

Safe foods

In order to find out what is safe for you to eat, we have to get you off all the foods which are potentially unsafe. In fact we have to clear these foods out of your body so completely that your body gets the chance to forget all about them. This is known as Phase I of the diet and takes about four weeks.

Phase I is strict because it is part of a test which you will complete in Phase II. Phase I should not leave you feeling hungry, but it does require you to abstain from foods which you may think of as staples, to shop for items which may seem unfamiliar and to spend a little time in the kitchen preparing them. But if you happen to have allergic water retention, Phase I brings rapid, almost instant weight loss. It is possible to lose up to 14 pounds in a week – but only if you don't cheat!

Testing foods

Next we have to reintroduce some of the omitted foods, one at a time, and observe in a very careful way how they affect you. This is known as Phase II of the diet and takes about four weeks. At the end of this time you will know which foods are safe for you to eat and which are unsafe.

Phase III follows Phase II and is permanent. In Phase III you resume a fairly normal diet, although if you want to prevent a return of your water retention, you will always have to be careful about consuming your unsafe foods. You will also need to keep on eating the beneficial foods which help to prevent water retention.

> **Caution**
>
> If you have been put on a special diet by a doctor or medical dietician and told that it could be dangerous for you to deviate from it, ask your doctor or dietician's advice before considering the Waterfall Diet.

The Waterfall Diet Phase I: What to eat

The 'yes' list consists of foods that you are allowed to eat in Phase I of the Waterfall Diet.

'Yes' List A: To eat as often as possible

- Fruit, especially dark-red and purple berries: blueberries, bilberries, blackberries, black cherries, black grapes and so on. Also oranges, pith from orange peel, lemons, lemon zest and pineapple. It is OK to cook fruit and eat it warm if you find it more filling this way. Fresh fruit is best, but frozen is OK too.
- Vegetables, especially brassicas, radishes and dark green, orange or purple vegetables: cabbage, Brussels sprouts, broccoli, kale, greens, carrots, pumpkin, red onions, beetroot (beets). Fresh is best, but frozen is OK too.
- Beans: aduki beans, mung beans, broad beans.
- Spices and flavourings: ginger, chives, garlic.
- Avocado pears.
- Celery, celery juice, parsley.

'Yes' List B: To eat in moderate amounts

- Wild or organically farmed fish and organically raised white meat such as chicken.

- All fruits and vegetables which are not in list A: e.g. cucumbers, watermelon, watercress, carrots, potatoes.
- Gluten-free grains and products such as breakfast cereals, crackers or snack bars that are made from them: brown rice, millet, maize (corn),* buckwheat, amaranth, quinoa.
- Low-gluten grains and products such as breakfast cereals, crackers or snack bars that are made from them: oats, barley, spelt, rye.**
- Olive oil (especially extra virgin) and soya oil.
- Nuts and seeds: e.g. Brazils, walnuts, sunflower seeds, sesame seeds, fresh natural peanuts.
- Other pulses or legumes which are not in list A: e.g. chickpeas, borlotti beans, lentils.
- Tofu and soy milk.*
- Herbs and spices and spice teas, especially chilli peppers, turmeric, cloves, black pepper, cinnamon, cardamom, fenugreek seeds, seaweed, garlic and ginger.
- Herbal teas, especially chamomile, fennel, peppermint.

'No' List: Foods to avoid completely

- Coffee.
- Sugar (including all sugar substitutes, honey, agave, syrup and foods or drinks containing added sugar).
- Salt.
- Highly salted or smoked foods and high-sodium items such as baking powder and baking soda. (*Salt substitutes are allowed but should be used sparingly; see p.192.*)

---

* A few people have an intolerance to soy products and maize. If any food on the 'yes' list seems to give you headaches or other troublesome symptoms, try to stop eating it to see if you feel better.
** Wheat is the most common problem grain, but some people are intolerant to other gluten-containing grains too. For best results, stick to gluten-free if you can.

- Fatty foods: red meat, pork, fatty meats, sausages and meat products, dips and sauces, potato crisps and chips, deep-fried foods, fried batter.
- White flour and products made from it.
- Alcohol.
- Artificial food additives, including sweeteners, preservatives, colourings and flavour enhancers.
- Wheat, as in bread, cake, biscuits, pasta, etc.
- Cow's milk products: milk, cheese, butter, yoghurt.
- Eggs (including foods containing traces of egg such as ice cream – read the labels!).
- Yeast (found mostly in baked products and alcoholic drinks).

Reasons for avoiding these foods, as well as useful substitutes to them, are listed on pages 197–201.

Foods that are on neither the 'yes' nor the 'no' list can be safely eaten in moderation, but to make sure, do check food labels for their ingredients. In general it's best to avoid convenience foods, as labels don't have to declare ingredients found within other ingredients. For instance, if you buy a packet food and it lists 'dried potato' as one of its ingredients, the label doesn't have to mention any preservatives which were included in the manufacture of the dried potato product.

   Try to stick as much as possible to using fresh, natural ingredients and cooking for yourself. Most of the recipes in this book are fairly quick and easy. You should not have to spend lots of time in the kitchen.

Special Waterfall Diet foods

Eat these as often as you can:

A. Blue and purple fruits

This includes blueberries, blackberries, bilberries, elderberries and black grapes. These fruits are the richest source of flavonoids, which help to keep your capillaries strong. Without enough flavonoids in your diet, capillaries can become fragile and leaky. This encourages water retention. Orange and lemon peel (including some of the white pithy part) are another good source of flavonoids.

B. Celery, celery juice and parsley

These are some of the richest sources of coumarin, a natural substance which is also found in grass and helps to give milk its rich flavour. Coumarin stimulates the immune system to break down protein particles which have escaped into the tissue spaces and lie there attracting excess fluid.

C. Almonds, sunflower and sesame seeds

Together with oats, oatmeal and leafy green vegetables, these are some of the best sources of magnesium, a mineral which is often lacking in the western diet but plays a vital role in the body's water balance. They also provide vitamin B_6 and zinc, which perform many tasks together with magnesium.

D. Broccoli, Brussels sprouts, cauliflower, cabbage and kale

These are not only rich in magnesium, they also help a woman's body to break down excessively high oestrogen levels which can encourage not just water retention, but PMS, fibroids, ovarian cysts and endometriosis. Broccoli stems can be juiced with a juice extractor.

E. Avocado pears

These are one of the richest sources of vitamin B_6. This vitamin is intimately involved in the production of hormones which help to control water balance, and it also aids the absorption of magnesium.

F. Warm food and warming spices (garlic, onion, chives, chilli, ginger, cardamom, fennel seeds, cinnamon, cloves)

Unless you live in a very warm part of the world, or unless you are a very hot-blooded athletic person, you may find that cold food and raw salads just don't fill you up or give you enough energy. In oriental medicine this type of food would be considered to encourage weight gain, as it depletes the body's 'fire' or yang energy. You will find hot lentil soup and casseroles flavoured with garlic, onion, chilli and ginger much more energising. Oriental experts believe that such foods burn off excess water in our bodies, and this is of course very good news for water retention sufferers. Don't overdo these spices. Burning your insides would be counter-productive and unnecessary. Another tip (if you can stand it!): do try to take a quick cold shower every morning. This really stimulates your metabolism.

G. Pineapple juice

A good source of bromelain (*see p.163*).

H. Natural diuretics

Cucumbers, watermelons, watercress, radishes (either small radishes or the long, white 'mooli' variety) lemons, cranberries, pomegranates, asparagus, carrots, celery seeds, fennel seeds and pumpkin seeds. A delicious diuretic drink can be made by extracting and mixing together the juices from cucumbers, radishes, carrots and celery. Whizz in some parsley before drinking. Leave radish juice to stand for at least 20 minutes before drinking otherwise the taste may be too peppery.

I. Aduki beans, mung beans, broad beans

In Chinese medicine these are considered to be very helpful in driving away water retention.

If any of the foods mentioned in this book are new to you, try consulting the staff at your local health food store. They will usually be delighted to help you find items such as celery juice and sunflower seeds, or to tell you how to make your own juices using a juice extractor machine. Also see pages 202–7 for advice on using selected alternatives.

7-day menu plan

All recipes can be found in the Recipes section starting on page 221. This is a suggested menu plan to get you started and give you ideas. This menu has been designed to ensure you get enough protein and special water-release foods, so if there's one food you don't like, make up for it by eating others from the same group instead. The groups are named A to G and are listed in the panel on page 176. So, for instance, if you dislike broccoli you can eat cabbage or Brussels sprouts instead, as they will do the same job. What will not work is to leave out a complete group altogether.

Monday

Breakfast

Wheat-free cereal* with cashew nuts and soya milk
Spice tea (*see below under Drinks*)
(*See more about breakfast on p.187.*)

Lunch

Aduki bean salad with parsley, chopped celery and French dressing, with rice or corn cake(s) or Ryvita and a scraping of pure olive oil spread

---

* *See panel on p.188.* You can also add fresh fruit or dried fruit such as raisins.

Hot broccoli soup with chives and parsley
A sliced orange, including some of the white pith

Dinner

Grilled or baked white fish with baked potato(es), braised vegetables and a sheep's yoghurt topping
Fresh or stewed blueberries with soya cream
A small glass of pineapple juice

Mid-evening

A small wineglass of fresh celery and radish juice
(Make this yourself: simply juice these vegetables with an electric juice extractor.)

Tuesday

Breakfast

Wheat-free cereal with soya milk and ground almonds
Spice tea

Lunch

Canned sardines in soya or olive oil, with rice or corn cake(s) or Ryvita and a scraping of pure olive oil spread
Hot broad bean soup with parsley
Black grapes

Dinner

Tofu, mushroom and broccoli stir-fry with rice noodles
Fresh tangerines with soya yoghurt and a little of the tangerine peel grated on top
A small glass of pineapple juice

Mid-evening

A small wineglass of fresh celery and radish juice

Wednesday

Breakfast

Wheat-free cereal with soya milk and ground sunflower seeds
Spice tea

Lunch

Hummus dip with rice or corn cake(s) or Ryvita
Hot watercress soup with chives and parsley
Fresh blueberries or black cherries

Dinner

Gluten-free pasta bake with chicken strips and vegetables
Fresh or canned (in natural juice) pineapple pieces with soya yoghurt
A small glass of fruit juice made from blueberries, blackberries or other dark red or purple fruit

Mid-evening

A small wineglass of fresh celery and radish juice

Thursday

Breakfast

Wheat-free cereal with soya milk and grated Brazil nuts (use a drum grater with a handle that you turn round)
Spice tea

Lunch

Goat's cheese on rice or corn cake(s) or Ryvita and a scraping of pure olive oil spread
Hot mung bean soup with ginger and parsley
A sliced orange, including some of the white pith

Dinner

Prawn Thai curry with brown rice and broccoli
A small glass of pineapple juice

Mid-evening

A small wineglass of fresh celery and radish juice

Friday

Breakfast

Wheat-free cereal with soya milk and chopped pumpkin seeds
Spice tea

Lunch

Rainbow salad with rice or corn cake(s) or Ryvita and a scraping of pure olive oil spread
Hot aduki bean soup with miso, ginger, parsley and arame
Black grapes

Dinner

Baked salmon parcels with new potatoes and cucumber salad
Exotic warm fruit salad in grape juice
A small glass of fruit juice made from blueberries, blackberries or other dark red or purple fruit

Mid-evening

A small wineglass of fresh celery and radish juice

Saturday

Brunch

Fried herring cakes with mushrooms and grilled tomatoes
Soya milk, banana and purple fruit smoothie
Spice tea

Dinner
   Broccoli soup with chives and parsley
   Red Thai curry with chicken, vegetables and rice noodles
   Brown rice pudding made with soya milk and cinnamon and
   topped with sugar-free black cherry jam
   A small glass of pineapple juice

Mid-evening
   A small wineglass of fresh celery and radish juice

Sunday

Brunch
   Kedgeree
   Soya milk, avocado and banana smoothie
   Spice tea

Dinner
   Hot broad bean soup with parsley
   Potato pancake with goat's cheese and spinach
   Black Forest gelled fruits with soya cream
   A small glass of pineapple juice

Mid-evening
   A small wineglass of fresh celery and radish juice

Drinks and snacks

Drinks
People with water retention need to drink water. Please ensure
that you consume at least two litres (eight US cups) of water a
day. The recommended herbal or spice teas can count towards this
if you wish.

Do not add sugar, honey, sweeteners or cow's milk to any drinks.

If you normally drink only tea and coffee, you may have come to believe that all your drinks should be brown! Naturally, this is not true. There are hundreds of good drinks waiting to be tried, though you may find it hard at first to break old habits.

All the following drinks are suitable for the Waterfall Diet. Home-made juices are concentrated plant nutrition in a glass, so they also have a highly therapeutic effect. You should try to drink at least one glass a day, especially of celery and radish juice.

You may have to look in a health food store to find some of the other suggested drinks.

Therapeutic drinks

- Home-made celery and radish juice. You can also add apple juice and parsley (*see p.273*).
- Spice tea, e.g. ginger, fennel or a proprietary brand such as Yogi tea with cinnamon, cloves, cardamom, etc. Try to add cinnamon whenever you can.
- Pineapple juice.
- Beetroot juice (either home-made or from a shop), mixed with celery and lemon juice (*see p.273*).
- Home-made broccoli stem and sharp apple juice (*see p.273*).
- Home-made flavonoid-rich orange juice (*see p.274*). Make it with a juice extractor rather than with a citrus juicer, and leave some of the white pith on the fruit.

Other fruit or vegetable juices

- Herbal teas: fennel, comfrey, chamomile, peppermint, nettle, parsley.

- Home-made clover tea: pick clover blossoms and dry them to bring out the coumarin.
- Plain water (preferably filtered or bottled).

Other drinks

- Fresh orange juice mixed with sparking mineral water.
- Iced herbal or rose-hip tea.
- Chicory or dandelion coffee with soya milk.
- Green tea (no more than two cups a week, as this is high in caffeine).
- Home-made fresh ginger tea with lemon zest. Add ground cinnamon, cloves and a little cayenne pepper, and this drink will help to prevent intestinal flatulence.

Snacks

These can be eaten if you need something between meals or if you are not hungry enough to eat a whole meal.

- Fruit, especially black grapes, berries, apples and oranges.
- Celery sticks, raw carrot sticks, radishes.
- A handful of Brazil nuts/sunflower seeds/almonds/cashew nuts.
- Home-roasted peanuts.
- Corn cakes, corn 'thins', corn crackers, rice cakes, Scottish oatcakes with nut butter or a scraping of pure olive oil spread and sugar-free jam.
- Any leftover dessert or breakfast items, or items from main meals which can be eaten cold.
- A bowl of hot vegetable soup.
- A pot of soya yoghurt (plain or with fruit pieces).
- Snack bars (*see the 'gluten-free' panel, p.188*).

Frequently asked questions

Q1. 'XYZ isn't on the 'yes' list. Can I eat it?'
A. Check the label for ingredients. If none of them are on the 'no' list, then you can eat it.

Q2. 'I am a vegetarian and don't eat chicken or fish. What can I eat instead?'
A. Be sure to include rice (or rice cakes) and nuts or tofu in every meal. One meal a day must also include beans or lentils. Don't try to skimp on this by eating more sheep or goat's cheese or yoghurt instead – even non-cow dairy items are deliberately kept in low quantities on the Waterfall Diet.

Q3. 'If I don't like or can't find an item on the 7-day menu, can I change it?'
A. As already mentioned, this menu has been designed to ensure you get enough protein and special water-release foods, so if there's one food you don't like you can make up for it by eating others from the same group instead. The groups are named A to G and are listed in the panel on page 176. So, for instance, if you dislike broccoli you can eat cabbage or Brussels sprouts instead, as they will do the same job. What will not work is to leave out a complete group altogether.

Q4. 'The recommended breakfasts are not enough to keep me going all morning. What can I add to them?'
A. You can add any of the items listed under 'Snacks', for instance corn thins or Scottish oatcakes with pure olive oil spread and sugar-free black cherry jam or crunchy peanut butter.

Q5. 'What if I'm not at home for Saturday brunch (for instance) and can't prepare the recommended meal?'
A. The order in which you eat the meals is not rigid. You can swap them around provided the balance of important items stays roughly the same.

Q6. 'This diet seems a bit monotonous, especially the drinks. Do I have to have pineapple juice, celery and radish juice every day?'
A. Other diets are based on controlling calories, fat, blood sugar and so on. The Waterfall Diet is a medical diet which aims to tackle the causes of water retention. It will work better if certain items are consumed every day. If you want, you can vary the times you consume them. This 7-day plan has been designed to be as quick and easy as possible. You can substitute some of the recipes starting on page 246 if you prefer, but do not leave out a complete food group (*see the panel on p.176*).

Q7. 'The menu plan doesn't state quantities. How do I know how much of each item I should eat?'
A. The Waterfall Diet does not aim to be calorie-controlled. The best advice is to eat sensible portion sizes that do not leave you feeling hungry. Unless you are an athlete or do a lot of manual labour, for most women this should add up to no more than 1,800 calories per day and for most men no more than 2,500 calories. If in doubt, check with a dietician. If you eat slowly you will find that you are satisfied more easily. The Waterfall Diet is based on healthy eating principles – the most important aspect of any diet.

Q8. 'I don't like the taste of the celery and radish juice. What can I do to improve it?'
A. Experiment with different flavours: try adding ingredients such as tomato, lemon or apple juice or a bit of chilli.

Q9. 'Since starting the Waterfall Diet I've been getting some symptoms which don't seem to be getting better.'
A. This occasionally happens when someone is allergic or intolerant to one of the foods allowed on Phase I of the diet. The most likely problem foods are soy products, corn and gluten, and occasionally peanuts or other nuts. Try eating a substitute for soy-based foods to see if the problem improves.

If that doesn't help, do the same with corn, or try going completely gluten free. It also helps if you keep a diary to help you pinpoint what you ate shortly before the symptoms developed.

After the first seven days
Continue for another three weeks to:

- Avoid even small amounts of foods on the 'no' list.
- Eat the foods on the 'yes' list.
- Consume the beneficial foods as frequently as possible.
- Balance foods by eating a good variety from each of the food groups listed in the panel on page 176.
- Use the same meal plan as for week 1 or try the additional recipes starting on page 246.

After you have been on Phase I for a total of four weeks, you can move on to Phase II in the next chapter.

Breakfast

Breakfast is the most important meal of the day, especially if you are dieting. When you sleep your body is fasting and its metabolism slows down. Eating a good breakfast stimulates your metabolism to speed up again, thus burning off your calories faster. Missing breakfast means keeping your metabolism slow until lunch time and will also leave you lacking in energy and feeling comparatively stressed and irritable.

Some people avoid breakfast because it leaves them feeling hungry again soon afterwards. This only happens when your breakfast consists mainly of carbohydrate, which sends your blood sugar up and then quickly down again, resulting in hunger. This is why the 7-day menu plan suggests that you sprinkle your breakfast cereal with chopped nuts.

Gluten-free products

Wheat is the most common problem grain, but some people are intolerant to other gluten-containing grains too. The Waterfall Diet is optionally gluten-free. Gluten-free grains include rice, millet, corn (maize), buckwheat, quinoa and amaranth.

Gluten-free breakfast cereals

Cornflakes and puffed rice should be gluten-free, but always check the label to make sure. Other gluten-free breakfast cereals can be found in health food stores and supermarkets. In the UK, larger branches of Sainsbury's now have several delicious varieties, including:

- Mesa Sunrise Indian corn, flax, and amaranth flakes (supplied by Nature's Path, www.naturespath.com)
- Toasted Buckwheat, Pumpkin Seed, Raisin and Mango breakfast mix
- Raisin, Almond, Mixed Seeds and Crispy Rice breakfast mix (supplied by Eat Natural, www.eatnatural.co.uk)
- Rice and Buckwheat cereal (supplied by Dove's Organic, www.dovesfarm.co.uk)
- Crushed Sunflower and Pumpkin Seeds or shelled hemp seeds (rich in protein and can be sprinkled on top of your cereal) (supplied by Virginia Harvest, www.virginiafoods.net)

Or, if you're in a hurry or just want a delicious snack:

- Wallaby bars, made from dried fruit, nuts and seeds (available from Holland and Barrett health food stores or online from www.healthlinkuk.com). For more information about Wallaby products, see www.energyproducts.com.au/productinfo.html

Gluten-free bread substitutes

(All are widely available in health food stores or supermarkets.)

- Rice cakes and corn thins (taste like popcorn) (supplied by Real Foods, www.realfoods.co.uk, though there are also many other brands of rice cakes)
- Corn cakes and corn crispbread (supplied by Orgran, www.orgran.com)
- Crispy Japanese rice cakes (supplied by Clearspring, www.clearspring.co.uk)

Gluten-free pasta substitutes

- Supplied by Orgran, www.orgran.com; other brands are also available

Gluten-free and sugar-free snack bars

- Wallaby bars (see above under 'Breakfast')

United States suppliers

In the US, brands which supply gluten-free foods include Nature's Path, Bob's Red Mill, Bakery on Main and U.S. Mills (Erewhon brand). For a wide selection of gluten-free products online, visit www.thebetterhealthstore.com or www.glutenfreemall.com. Many local health food stores sell a good selection.

Australian suppliers

Orgran is an Australian brand and markets many gluten-free products. Wallaby bars also come from Australia.

Useful hints and tips for getting through Phase I

Getting started

Don't start the Waterfall Diet until you are properly organised. If you shop weekly in a supermarket, check that it can provide everything you need. If not, ask in your local health food store. If trying to save money, buy your fish and vegetables from a fishmonger and greengrocer – they will be cheaper. Check the availability of organic chicken and vegetables from your local organic supplier, or see Useful Addresses on page 276 for national suppliers.

Check that the diet will work into your schedule. If you usually come home hungry after working late and grab something quick from the fridge, you will need to make sure that it's going to be compatible with this diet.

Make lots of thick bean and vegetable stews to keep in the fridge to heat up quickly when you get home – or put them in a 'slow cooker' so that delicious smells will waft through the door to greet you. Cook a large pan of brown rice and when cold freeze it in portions ready for defrosting and quickly heating up when needed. Do the same with a packet of dried peas or beans. Since you will probably need packed lunches if you go out to work, organise these the night before, and buy a Thermos so that you can take hot soup with you.

Proper preparations will make the Waterfall Diet much easier and more enjoyable. The first week is the most difficult time; if you can get through that you will probably succeed and reap all the benefits which the diet brings. You may lose not only your water retention but a host of minor problems such as sleeping difficulties, headaches, spotty skin, constipation, bloating, sore joints, premenstrual symptoms and lack of energy.

Equipment

Although not vital, you will find it much easier to follow the Waterfall Diet if you have access to a freezer and a pressure cooker.

The latter is especially good for dried pulses, because it can cook them in a few minutes whereas ordinary boiling can take hours. Do also try to get a juice extractor, since otherwise you will not be able to make the juices that will help you so much by extracting concentrated nutrients from celery, radishes and other fruit and vegetables.

'I haven't got time to cook!'

Everyone has time to cook, but not everyone makes cooking a priority! Most of us have also got out of the habit of regular cooking because it is so much easier to buy ready-made foods.

With the Waterfall Diet, an hour or two spent in the kitchen can result in mountains of food ready for freezing or storing in the fridge for instant use over the next few days. For instance, a large pan of soup will last four or five days, a bag of frozen brown rice will give you up to half a dozen meals, and a bag of frozen beans will provide masses of great-value instant protein.

Just stir-fry tofu with some olive oil, herbs, pepper and garlic, add cooked fresh vegetables, and you will have a meal far cheaper and just as quick as anything you can buy ready-made, but with far more health benefits. Or pop some frozen butter beans (lima beans) into a large pan of cooked, liquidised carrots, potatoes, leeks and onions, heat through and add soya cream. What could be simpler and more delicious?

A frozen fillet of sole takes minutes to defrost in hot water and then grill or broil. You can also make liberal use of frozen vegetables and leftover fresh vegetables. In fact why not make a point of cooking more vegetables than you need so that you have enough to last you for a few days, heated up with steamed potato pieces in a tightly lidded pan with some olive oil and a few tablespoons of water. Serve with your grilled fish.

Check labels carefully

Most commercial foods have a habit of including small amounts of wheat, egg, yeast or dairy produce in the small print, so do make sure you study labels on packets before buying, and if you don't know what terms like 'modified starch' or 'casein' mean, assume that to be on the safe side you can't have them. Home-made is best, since you know exactly what you have put into each dish.

Gluten-free foods

Health food stores and most larger supermarkets now have shelves dedicated to gluten-free products. Some of these products are also free of eggs and cow's milk, and so are suitable for the Waterfall Diet. This is where you can find items like gluten-free pasta, rice milk (the 'Rice Dream' brand is delicious) and corn cakes or corn thins which have the delicious taste of popcorn (*see p.189*).

Salt substitutes

These can be found in larger health food stores or online. 'No Salt' (from Prewett) or 'Salt Rite' (in the UK) and 'Also Salt' or 'Morton Salt' (in the US) are salt substitutes but should be used sparingly.

Getting enough calcium

Since Phase I of the Waterfall Diet does not allow cow's milk or dairy produce, your friends and family could become concerned that you might not get enough calcium, particularly if you are worried about preventing brittle bone disease (osteoporosis). Some doctors and dieticians, too, may try to pressurise you into consuming milk and cheese because these are the easiest ways to obtain this essential mineral. If in doubt, contact the Vegan Society (*see Useful Addresses on p.276*), which can provide scientific information written by qualified state-registered dieticians on the health and safety of dairy-free diets.

Almonds and carob flour are a rich source of calcium, followed by dark-green leafy vegetables like kale and broccoli, and sunflower or sesame seeds, Brazil nuts and tofu.

Getting enough protein

As you know, a protein deficiency can encourage water retention, so it is important to eat enough protein every day. The menu plans suggested for the Waterfall Diet take this into account, but if you try to adapt them, remember that you must consume good portions of the following foods every day: nuts or seeds (e.g. sunflower seeds), pulses (e.g. beans, lentils, tofu or soya flour), brown rice and fish or organic chicken. Don't get stuck on just one or two of these for convenience's sake; most plant proteins are not complete proteins. You need as much variety as possible.

Coping with sugar cravings

These cravings can be hard to cope with, especially when you are not allowed artificial sweeteners either. Sugary foods tend to be our 'comfort' foods. In avoiding them we feel we are being deprived of comfort as well as enjoyment.

So you will be very pleased to know that the most harmful effect of sugar consumption – its tendency to raise insulin levels too quickly and too high – can be largely prevented if you eat naturally sweet foods rather than foods with added sugar. This is because the natural sugars in these foods are bound tightly to the dietary fibre they contain and the digestive process cannot separate the two very quickly. This results in a slower absorption of sugar and a more gradual rise in insulin levels.

Naturally sweet foods include apples, oranges, bananas, sultanas, dates, dried apricots and other dried fruit, but honey and natural syrups are not permitted since these have a similar effect on your metabolism to ordinary sugar.

If you sweeten your snacks and desserts with naturally sweet foods, you will hardly notice that you are unable to eat sugar.

Coping with chocolate cravings

While it is an acquired taste, a craving for chocolate may have started with an attempt by your body to get more of the minerals magnesium and iron, which are found in cocoa powder. Since the Waterfall Diet provides healthy amounts of both minerals, it should help you to lose any physical addiction to chocolate. This just leaves the psychological cravings of comfort eating!

The best way to deal with this is to eat or drink something else which makes you feel that you have had a treat. Alternatively, make yourself a delicious chocolate banana cream boat using the recipe on page 250. Using only a little cocoa powder, it will give you the taste of chocolate without the excess fat and sugar, and will help with that element of comfort. I also like to whisk a little cocoa powder into a cup of warm Rice Dream.

Treats don't have to be edible – you could buy yourself something new to wear, or have a new hairdo, or do something special that you have been promising yourself for years but never got around to: learning to ride a horse or a motorbike, planning a Caribbean cruise or taking up a creative new hobby. You may soon have a brand-new figure to do it in!

Coping with business lunches, restaurants and dining out

Many business executives feel very pressured to be 'one of the lads' when it comes to wining and dining. But the truth is that most of the business world is becoming increasingly health-conscious and you may well find that your client or host is also on a diet. Brazen it out and explain that your diet is just temporary. Tell them about it. They may even want to join you in adopting it!

Opting for mineral water, grilled fish or roast chicken and vegetables, followed by fruit, is usually possible in most restaurants. Ethnic restaurants often offer plain rice and vegetable or lentil dishes, rice noodles, tofu, fish and other non-meat options, though beware monosodium glutamate (MSG) in Chinese sauces, and a possibly excessive use of soy sauce, which is high in salt. Japanese sushi is often compatible with the Waterfall Diet.

As far as dining out is concerned, do tell your friends that you are on a diet and let anyone who is going to cook for you have a list of permitted ingredients. They may well be very interested and keen to accommodate you. Perhaps they will want to take up the diet themselves!

I am sometimes asked, 'What can I do if, due to completely unforeseen circumstances, there is absolutely nothing suitable for me to eat?' Some of the least harmful occasional sins during Phase I of this diet would include ordinary fried or roast chicken (no coating), French fries, white rice (but not white bread or other wheat-containing food), fried fish with the coating removed and a little red meat: beef and pork.

Drinks

Tea, coffee, cola and beer are not essentials – water is! Drinking water in preference to other drinks helps to dilute the fluid in your tissue spaces; as explained in Chapter 7, the more dilute it is, the more easily it can get back into your blood capillaries. While tap water contains a lot of chlorine and other impurities, bottled water can work out quite expensive, so you may want to invest in a water filter.

Using canned and frozen foods

These foods can be great time-savers, but must comply with the general rules of the Waterfall Diet. So in Phase I, where products containing sugar are not allowed, you would not be able to eat fruit preserved in syrup (which is made from sugar), but plain frozen fruit or fruit canned or bottled in its own juice is the next best thing to fresh. Likewise, frozen vegetables or Italian plum tomatoes canned in their own juice are fine, but try to avoid brands containing artificial additives. Other types of canned vegetables are probably high in salt and should be avoided. Do remember that, while convenience is sometimes important, fresh is always best for your body, because the longer food is stored, the more nutrients like vitamin C and some of the B vitamins are destroyed.

Coping with side-effects from the Waterfall Diet

Most people are likely to experience side-effects from the Waterfall Diet – usually caffeine withdrawal symptoms in the form of a nagging headache for a day or two. If it becomes difficult to cope with, take plain aspirin (the cheap kind, not 'soluble' or 'dispersible', as these contain additives), but try not to take paracetamol (acetaminophen) or other painkillers since these are usually more stressful for your liver.

Other potential side-effects are weakness and fatigue if you do not eat enough calories. Don't try to kill two birds with one stone by also turning this into a very low-calorie diet. If you don't eat enough calories then instead of concentrating on the long-term adjustments to your eating habits that you must make after Phases I and II to keep your water retention away, you will just be desperate to come off this diet and resume eating all the foods that were giving you water retention.

Remember that to keep up your calorie intake, you will probably need to eat more food than usual on the Waterfall Diet – especially for breakfast and lunch. Although you may have been used to no more than a cup of coffee and a sandwich, with a couple of bars of chocolate in between, the calories in a bar of chocolate can be the equivalent of a whole meal on the Waterfall Diet!

If you are not used to eating a fibre-rich diet like the Waterfall Diet, you may react with more wind or looser bowel motions than usual. It will settle down eventually. Drinking strong spice tea with meals is very effective at reducing gas. Eat little and often for the time being, and avoid eating large amounts of any particularly 'windy' foods.

'What if I just can't get to grips with the diet and want to give up?'

The recommended time to spend on Phase I is four weeks. This gives your body time to carry out some repair work on the damage caused by previous faulty eating habits or by special nutritional needs going unfulfilled. But if you feel that you can't cope with four weeks, set yourself a target of two weeks instead. If you want to give up after two weeks and move on to Phase II, you can, and, although it's not ideal, you will still have received some benefits. On the other hand, most people find that after managing for two weeks they have got over most of the problems and the rest is plain sailing. You might even find that it takes a couple of practice runs to get into it, so don't lose heart. If you can't manage the full four weeks the first time, try again later on.

Reasons for the 'no' list of foods
More information about the suggested alternatives is given on pages 202–7.

Food	Coffee
Reason for avoidance	Diuretic effect. Can make Type II water retention worse by dehydrating your blood. Coffee also causes loss of magnesium and other minerals and increases your liver's workload.
Alternatives	Chicory and dandelion coffee
Food	Sugar, honey, agave, syrup, and foods containing added sugar. Read your labels, since sugar is also known as *sucrose, glucose, dextrose and fructose.*
Reason for avoidance	Sugar is absorbed into your blood and turned into glucose much more quickly than any other foods. This can make your insulin levels rise too quickly and too high. High insulin levels make you retain sodium (and water) and encourage fatty deposits in arteries and as stored body fat, especially around your middle! Large amounts of sugar also seem to have a harmful effect on the kidneys and can cause them to become enlarged (*see p.38*). Like fat, sugar is very high in calories yet contains no nutrients of its own. It therefore 'dilutes' your diet, resulting in an overall decrease in vitamins and minerals and other important nutrients which help to prevent water retention. Honey and syrup have similar effects on hormones – they are still concentrated forms of sugar. Agave is mostly fructose, which can raise levels of fats in your blood.
Alternatives	Use naturally sweet foods like bananas, raisins and dates.

Table continued ▶

Reasons for the 'no' list of foods
More information about the suggested alternatives is given on pages 202–7.

Food	Fat, especially saturated fat, in large amounts as found in fatty minced beef and burgers, sausages, pork pies, chocolate, crisps, fried food, butter, margarine, cream and cheese, mayonnaise, pastry, and many sauces, dips and desserts made from these.
Reason for avoidance	Fat is not a poison and does not need to be avoided completely. In fact it is essential to have some fat (in the form of essential polyunsaturated oils) in your diet. But by consuming far too much of the foods listed opposite, most of us eat far more fat than we realise since the fat in these foods is mostly invisible. 　　A diet which contains a lot of high-fat foods can encourage water retention in several ways: 1. In time it may impair kidney function. 2. It will also encourage deficiencies of nutrients needed for strong capillary walls, since it is high in calories yet contains few nutrients of its own. Like sugar, fat 'dilutes' your overall diet. 3. Animal fat contains arachidonic acid, which can encourage inflammation in your skin, joints or other parts of your body, and therefore water retention.
Alternatives	(to saturated fat) Oils, especially extra virgin olive oil and unrefined sunflower or soya oil. Also nuts and seeds used in meals will provide the essential polyunsaturated oils that your body needs and will help to make a meal filling.
Food	1. Salt, and highly salted or smoked foods such as salami, ham and bacon, smoked fish, salty cheeses, stock cubes, yeast extract, soy sauce and ready prepared pies, tarts, sauces, or commercially made 'oven-ready' dishes. 2. Sodium-rich drinks, medicines and food additives. Baking powder. Most commercial soft drinks are very high in sodium. Some medicines, such as antacids based on bicarbonate of soda or effervescent tablets of any kind, can also contain large amounts of sodium. One of the most common food additives is a flavour-enhancer known as mono*sodium* glutamate or 'E621'. Other sodium-rich food additives are E211, E223, E250, E251, E262(ii), E281, E339, E350, E401, E452, E466, E500, E514, E524, R541, E576.

Reasons for the 'no' list of foods

More information about the suggested alternatives is given on pages 202–7.

Reason for avoidance	There is a direct relationship between the amount of salt or sodium you consume and the amount of water you retain. Reducing your salt or sodium consumption will *immediately* result in some loss of retained fluid since water always follows sodium.
	Since the UK Food Standards Agency recently announced that manufacturers were putting too much salt in our food, many processed foods, such as bread, ready-meals, commercial vegetable juices and so on now contain less. This is good news, but most of us are *still* consuming far too much salt for good health.
Alternatives	Salt substitutes, miso, a Japanese paste made from fermented soya, low-sodium baking powder. To help with flavouring, a small amount of tamari sauce (wheat-free soy sauce) is included in some of the recipes. Miso and tamari sauce are not sodium-free, but a little goes a long way.
Food	White flour
Reason for avoidance	White flour is often more enjoyable than wholemeal in foods like cakes, biscuits, doughnuts, sauces, pastry and pasta. Some people also prefer it in bread. But it cannot be emphasised enough that white flour is almost devoid of many important minerals like magnesium and zinc, and is so poor in B vitamins that by law some of the ones you may not easily get elsewhere in your diet have to be artificially replaced! Once you have reduced your water retention, by all means have some foods made from white flour if your type of water retention permits it, but remember that the more of them you eat, the more you risk inadequately nourishing your body and so damaging its performance.
	White flour is also a very poor source of dietary fibre, which is needed to prevent constipation. (*See p.72 for some of the important reasons for avoiding constipation.*)
Alternatives	Brown rice flour is light in colour and texture and can be used in baking if recipes are adapted to take into account its lack of gluten. Some health stores are now selling gluten-free flour which can be used in white flour recipes and is made from barley, rice, millet and maize.

Table continued ▶

Reasons for the 'no' list of foods
More information about the suggested alternatives is given on pages 202–7.

Food	Alcohol
Reason for avoidance	Alcohol blocks anti-diuretic hormone (ADH), a hormone which slows down urination when your body's fluid levels are getting low. So alcohol makes you lose more fluid even when you are *already* dehydrated. As mentioned above, dehydration is especially undesirable if you suffer from Type II water retention and can make it worse.
Alternatives	See the suggested drinks on page 183.

Food	Artificial food additives
Reason for avoidance	It is hard to avoid these if we eat commercially manufactured foods. Almost everything contains a cocktail of additives: preservatives, colourings, artificial sweeteners, flavourings and flavour enhancers, to name just a few. Sometimes the law does not even require additives to be listed on a packet. For instance a chilled meal purchased from a supermarket may appear to contain no additives at all, but this is because items like 'stock' do not have to declare small amounts of sub-ingredients they contain.
	The problem with additives is that we only know if they harm the health of well-nourished laboratory animals given them singly in large quantities. We have no idea how they affect the health of humans when consumed over a lifetime in dozens of different combinations.
	Some additives are known to trigger problems like asthma and skin rashes in children. Others have been banned *after* it was discovered that they were unsafe. One thing we do know is that your liver must try to break down these foreign chemicals and uses up its precious resources in doing so. What we do not know is how successful *your* liver is in coping and whether it forms any toxic intermediate products which linger in your system and cause damage which may encourage water retention (*see p.81*).
Alternatives	There are now many additive-free products on the market. Health food stores often specialise in them. Or make your own additive-free food.

Reasons for the 'no' list of foods
More information about the suggested alternatives is given on pages 202–7.

Food	Potential allergens: wheat (and bread, pasta, etc., made from wheat), dairy produce, eggs and yeast
Reason for avoidance	Almost all people who suffer from the kind of food intolerance which leads to water retention (*see Chapter 2*) will improve if they avoid these four foods. So Phase I of the Waterfall Diet excludes these foods to help you release any fluid which they may have been causing. You will be testing them one by one in Phase II to see if any particular one brings a return of your water retention.
Alternatives	To wheat: Spelt, rice, barley, rye, millet flour, etc. To milk: Soya milk, nut milk, rice milk. To eggs: In cakes, a mixture of soya flour and soya milk can often replace eggs due to the high protein content. To bread made with yeast: Yeast- and wheat-free pumpernickel (black rye bread). Rice, corn or rye cakes or crackers or crispbreads. To stock cubes and gravy mixes containing yeast: Miso, which has a savoury flavour and can be dissolved in water.
Food	Red meat of all types and non-organically farmed white meat
Reason for avoidance	Red meat (even if apparently lean) and saturated fat contain arachidonic acid, which can encourage inflammation in your skin, joints or other parts of your body, and thus water retention. White meat (poultry) is much less fatty and so less likely to be a problem, but please avoid it during Phase I of the diet unless it has been organically raised. Even free-range chickens may be fed standard commercial feed which contains antibiotics, dung from other chickens and other unsavoury items. We do not know how well a chicken's liver can cope with these challenges and what kind of residues remain in the bird's meat and fat. Although not related to water retention, it is important for your general health to know that non-organic chickens are routinely fed antibiotics, that bacteria in the chicken's intestines can become resistant to them and that bacteria in humans who consume the birds can acquire this resistance. This has led to life-threatening cases where salmonella poisoning, for instance, becomes virtually untreatable because no antibiotic is effective.
Alternatives	Fish, organically-raised white meat, tofu.

If it seems that all your favourite foods are forbidden, don't worry. Phase I of the Waterfall Diet only lasts for four weeks and its benefits start very quickly. Meanwhile, there are lots of delicious alternatives, and while you are spending the first few weeks trying them out, you will gradually miss your old favourites less and less.

Using unfamiliar ingredients

Ingredient	Aduki beans and mung beans
Where to get it	Health food stores, Asian grocery stores
What it's good for	According to Chinese medicine, these beans help to drive off water retention.
How to use it	Like other beans, these small beans need to be soaked overnight before cooking. Drain, add fresh water then boil fast for ten minutes before simmering for 30 to 40 minutes until tender. After cooling can be spread out and frozen.

Ingredient	Alfalfa sprouts
Where to get it	Health food stores (seeds also sold)
What it's good for	Rich in coumarin.
How to use it	Add to salads or use as a garnish like cress. Alfalfa sprouts or seeds can be bought in packets from health food stores. To sprout the seeds yourself, place a level tablespoon of seeds in a large jar, then cover the jar with a piece of nylon fabric from an old pair of tights and secure the fabric with an elastic band around the neck of the jar. Run some water into the jar, shake to thoroughly wet the seeds, then leave overnight. In the morning, pour the water away, straining it through the nylon cover. Every morning and night, rinse the seeds by pouring in water and immediately straining it out again, and in a few days you will have a luscious growth of curly green sprouts which can be added to soups or eaten as salad. Eat them when they are about 1 inch (2.5 cm) long. You can also follow the same procedure to sprout lentils, mung beans, aduki beans, black buckwheat grains, barley grains and clover seeds.

Ingredient	Bilberries
Where to get it	Frozen food departments of some larger supermarkets
What it's good for	Rich in flavonoids.
How to use it	Allow to defrost, then consume them as they are, or place in an oven-proof casserole dish in a medium oven for 25 minutes or until the fruits split and the juices run. Serve hot or cold, with soya cream, or combine with gelatine or vegetarian gelling product before cooling to make bilberry jelly. If sweetening is required, use a small amount of puréed dates.

Using unfamiliar ingredients

Ingredient	Blueberries
Where to get it	Fruit departments of some larger supermarkets. Some health shops may also sell sugar-free blueberry jam.
What it's good for	Rich in flavonoids.
How to use it	Serve fresh with soya yoghurt, or cook as for bilberries. Should need no sweetening as blueberries are sweeter than bilberries.
	Use sugar-free blueberry jam as any other jam.

Ingredient	Brown rice
Where to get it	Supermarkets and health food shops
What it's good for	Rich in B vitamins.
How to use it	Brown rice is nuttier and has a different texture from white rice. Wash thoroughly, then pre-soak overnight in at least twice its volume of filtered water. Before cooking, drain the water away and add fresh water to cover the rice generously. Bring to the boil then cover tightly and simmer on the lowest possible heat for 20–25 minutes. Bite one of the grains to check that the rice is tender. Strain quickly with a sieve, replace the rice in the saucepan, cover then leave the rice to steam in the covered pan away from the heat for 5 minutes, after which it is ready to serve.
	Once cold, brown rice can be spread out on an oiled baking tray, frozen, then crumbled into grains and bagged for the freezer.

Ingredient	Buckwheat
Where to get it	Health food shops
What it's good for	Rich in magnesium and in the flavonoid rutin, which helps to build capillary strength.
How to use it	Buckwheat is a gluten-free grain unrelated to wheat and is a good alternative for wheat- and gluten-allergy sufferers. The grains can be cooked like rice, or are available as a flour, which is the main ingredient of small Russian pancakes known as blinis.
	To cook buckwheat grains, soak overnight in twice their volume of water, then bring to the boil and simmer very gently with the lid on for 15–20 minutes, or until the grains are tender. Use as an alternative to rice.

Ingredient	Carob flour
Where to get it	Health food shops
What it's good for	Very rich in calcium. Naturally sweet and often used as a healthier alternative to chocolate.
How to use it	The carob is a type of bean. It is made into flour which can be incorporated in cakes and biscuits to give a light brown colour and natural sweetness.

Table continued ▶

Using unfamiliar ingredients

Ingredient	Dandelion coffee
Where to get it	Health food stores
What it's good for	Helps to drain the liver and gall bladder.
How to use it	Can be bought as granules and used as instant coffee. If you find it lacks flavour, try mixing it with chicory coffee.

Ingredient	Dried beans (large), split peas, chickpeas, marrowfat peas
Where to get it	Supermarkets, grocers' and health food stores
What it's good for	A very cheap source of protein, rich in dietary fibre.
How to use it	These should be soaked in water before use. Cover with four times their volume in boiling filtered water and leave overnight. Throw away the soaking water, place the beans, just covered with fresh water, in a pressure cooker, bring to full steam, and cook for 3–10 minutes, depending on size and age. Pressure-cooking breaks down the poisonous lectins found in raw beans. If you do not have a pressure cooker, boil them fast for at least 10 minutes before simmering or slow-cooking. Conventional boiling can take an hour or more to soften them, depending on age and size. To freeze, allow to cool and follow the same procedure as for brown rice (*see above*).

Ingredient	Gluten-free pasta
Where to get it	Supermarkets and health food stores
What it's good for	Alternatives to wheat pasta.
How to use it	These very useful products help to make a quick meal. There are many different varieties made from grains such as rice, millet and buckwheat. Use just like normal pasta.

Ingredient	Herbal teas and spice teas
Where to get it	Health food stores
What it's good for	Often rich in flavonoids, coumarin or other beneficial ingredients. Spice teas contain 'warming' ingredients which, according to Chinese medicine, help to drive off water retention.
How to use it	Some beneficial herbal teas are buckwheat, chamomile, clover blossom, nettle, parsley and fennel teas, or a mixture of any of these. Beneficial spice teas include cinnamon, ginger, cloves, cardamom, or a mixture of any of these.

Ingredient	Lentils (red, green, brown, puy and other varieties)
Where to get it	Lentils are widely available, but health food stores and ethnic shops tend to provide the most choice of varieties.
What it's good for	Rich in protein and dietary fibre.
How to use it	Use to make lentil curry (dahl) or soup. No pre-soaking required. Lentils take 20–30 minutes to cook, depending on size.

Using unfamiliar ingredients

Ingredient	Low-sodium baking powder
Where to get it	Health food stores or online
What it's good for	Allows you to bake cakes, scones and biscuits without the high sodium levels found in ordinary baking powder.
How to use it	Use in accordance with the manufacturer's directions on the container.

Ingredient	Miso
Where to get it	Health food stores and some larger supermarkets
What it's good for	Dark brown stock paste. Unlike most stock paste, miso is very rich in vitamins and minerals and lower in sodium. It also contains protein.
How to use it	Mix with boiling water and use to make gravy and to flavour dark soups and stews. One variety of miso is made with wheat and should be avoided during Phases I and II of the Waterfall Diet. (Always check the list of ingredients on the label first.) Other types, such as barley miso, are OK. Don't overdo the miso – it does contain salt. Use just enough to get some colour and flavour into a dish.

Ingredient	Oats
Where to get it	Widely available. Health food shops sell organically grown oats
What it's good for	Rich in B vitamins, magnesium and dietary fibre.
How to use it	Make rolled oats into porridge for breakfast, or soak oatmeal in water overnight and add soya milk in the morning to make a creamy muesli. Oats are also used to make flapjacks and oat biscuits and are found in cereal snack bars.

Ingredient	Olive oil spread
Where to get it	Widely available in health food stores and supermarkets
What it's good for	Good alternative to butter and margarine.
How to use it	Pure olive oil spread simply consists of olive oil which has been solidified and made spreadable. The brand I use is Belazu.

Ingredient	Pumpernickel bread
Where to get it	Supermarkets, health food stores
What it's good for	Wholegrain rye bread with a sweetish, nutty flavour. Buy a brand which contains no yeast or wheat.
How to use it	Eat with soups and salads, or make into an open sandwich (to eat with a knife and fork) by spreading with hummus and adding salad toppings or alfalfa sprouts.

Table continued ▶

Using unfamiliar ingredients

Ingredient	Salt substitutes
Where to get it	Health food stores, supermarkets and online
What it's good for	Allows you to season your food without high levels of sodium. May also increase valuable potassium.
How to use it	Add to food as you would ordinary salt. 'Low-sodium' salt products consist of half to two-thirds potassium salt and the rest ordinary sodium salt or sea salt. Even better, some suppliers now sell sodium-free salt (*see p.192*).

Ingredient	Seaweed
Where to get it	Health food stores
What it's good for	One of the very few good sources of iodine.
How to use it	Use a few strands of arame seaweed in soups.

Ingredient	Sheep's milk yoghurt
Where to get it	Supermarkets, health-food stores
What it's good for	An alternative to cow's milk yoghurt.
How to use it	Use as normal yoghurt.

Ingredient	Soya cream
Where to get it	Supermarkets, health-food stores
What it's good for	A blend of soya protein and oil which can be used as an alternative to dairy single cream.
How to use it	Soya cream is used as a topping for desserts, or can be stirred into soup or gravy to achieve the same effect as single cream. Look for it under brand names such as Provamel's 'Soya Dream'.

Ingredient	Soya flour
Where to get it	Health food stores. Try to get an organic brand or a brand which avoids buying from suppliers who grow genetically modified crops.
What it's good for	High in protein. Provides all the benefits of soy foods, including protection against prostate cancer and menopausal problems.
How to use it	A few tablespoons of soya flour can often be used as an alternative to eggs in baking because of its high protein content.

Ingredient	Soya milk
Where to get it	Widely available. (*See note under Soya flour.*)
What it's good for	Provides all the benefits of soy foods.
How to use it	Use in the same way as cow's milk. Contains less protein, calcium and fat, but a good balance of vitamins and minerals. Some brands are enriched with calcium. Cook slowly with brown rice to make great rice pudding.

Using unfamiliar ingredients

Ingredient	Soya yoghurt
Where to get it	Supermarkets and health food stores. If you have difficulty finding it, ask for plain Yofu or Sojasun, which is a good thick brand. Or make your own (*see recipe on p.269*). (*See note under Soya flour.*)
What it's good for	An alternative to cow's milk yoghurt. Provides all the benefits of soy foods, plus the friendly bacteria found in normal yoghurt.
How to use it	Use as normal yoghurt.

Ingredient	Spelt flour
Where to get it	Health food stores and some supermarkets
What it's good for	An alternative to wholewheat flour, also known as 'ancient wheat'. Many people who are allergic to wheat are not allergic to spelt.
How to use it	Use exactly as wholewheat flour. You can also buy pasta made from spelt.

Ingredient	Sugar-free jam
Where to get it	Some larger supermarkets and superstores sell the excellent St Dalfour brand.
What it's good for	The blueberry and black cherry varieties of this jam are rich in flavonoids.
How to use it	Use as normal jam.

Ingredient	Sugar-free marmalade
Where to get it	Health food stores. Also St Dalfour Thick Cut Orange Spread.
What it's good for	Citrus peel is rich in flavonoids and coumarin.
How to use it	Use as normal marmalade.

Ingredient	Tamari sauce
Where to get it	Health food shops
What it's good for	A type of soy sauce, made without using wheat.
How to use it	Use tamari sauce sparingly (it is salty), to flavour stir-fried dishes. For dark soups and sauces use wheat-free miso (*see above*).

Ingredient	Tofu
Where to get it	Supermarkets and health food stores. (*See note under Soya flour.*)
What it's good for	A good source of protein made from soy – as good as eating meat but with added health benefits.
How to use it	'Silken' tofu is good for liquidising and making into mayonnaise, 'cheese'-cake, or layering with vegetables, etc., in oven-baked vegetable dishes. Ordinary firm tofu is best for cutting into cubes, dusting with brown rice flour and frying in oil. Can be marinated beforehand.

CHAPTER 13

Phase II of the Waterfall Diet: What foods are safe for you to eat?

Phase II of the Waterfall Diet also takes four weeks. It is similar to Phase I, but is in fact a four-week self-test. This test involves reintroducing one at a time some of the foods left out of Phase I to see if they bring a return of your water retention or of any other symptoms that got better during Phase I. Once you have completed Phase II, you will know which foods are safe for you to eat and which (if any) were contributing to your water retention. When foods cause water retention or other unpleasant symptoms, you are said to be 'intolerant' to these foods.

Phase I must be carried out first before you can proceed to Phase II. You cannot expect to get any answers by carrying out Phase II on its own. This is because your body has to be completely clear of all suspect foods for several weeks.

As explained in Chapter 2, a lot of water retention can be caused by an intolerance or 'allergy' to common foods. But if these are foods you eat several times every day, you will never get the chance to associate them with your problem. You will just have water retention, which might be a little better in the mornings when you have not eaten for a while.

The foods which most people eat very frequently are some of the main ones on your 'no' list:

- Wheat (found in bread, flour, cakes, pasta, pizza, etc.).
- Dairy products (found in milk, cream, cheese, yoghurt, butter and anything containing these).
- Yeast (found in alcoholic drinks, stock cubes and other savoury flavourings, gravy mix, bread and pizza).
- Egg (found in egg dishes, egg pasta, many brands of ice-cream, desserts, batter, pancakes, etc.).

If you lost more than a couple of pounds of fluid within a few days during Phase I of the Waterfall Diet, it is almost certainly because you were avoiding these four food groups.

In Phase II we are going to introduce these foods one at a time in a very controlled way, to find out which ones are safe for you to eat and which ones were contributing to your water retention. This type of test is known as the 'avoidance and challenge test'. That's because you avoid a suspect food for four weeks and then challenge yourself by re-introducing it and noting down any effects it has.

Some practitioners recommend blood tests to identify problem foods or food intolerances. I have sometimes arranged these tests for clients, but they can work out quite expensive and I never completely trust them. The most reliable type (known as the ELISA test) analyses whether different foods cause a certain type of antibody to be formed in your blood. The presence of the antibody suggests that you are allergic or intolerant to that food.

The reason why I don't trust these tests is that food is never supposed to come into contact with your blood. Before it is absorbed into your blood, it should be broken down by enzymes in your intestines into sugars, amino acids and fatty acids, individual vitamins, etc. No trace of the original food should remain. Undigested food particles can only get into your blood if your intestinal wall is damaged. The usual kind of damage involved here is 'leaky gut syndrome', as discussed earlier. When someone has this condition, almost anything they eat is liable to attract the antibodies which a blood test looks for. The problem is not the food itself, but how well it has been digested and the condition of the intestine. So a positive result does not necessarily mean that the food in question is responsible for the water retention.

The avoidance and challenge test, overleaf, which you will be using for the next four weeks is reliable because you can clearly see for yourself any association between the foods you eat and your symptoms or water retention.

Apart from rapid weight gain, examples of some of the reactions you should note down are: drowsiness, headaches, joint pains or tenderness, skin rashes or itching, bloating, gas, tummy pains, diarrhoea, constipation, coughing, wheezing and heartburn. Any foods which seem to provoke any of these reactions are unsafe foods for you.

If you are not completely sure about the results for any one of these foods:

- Finish all four tests.
- Continue avoiding all four food groups for another week.
- Repeat the test for the suspect food.

Once you have completed all these tests, and have made a note of your unsafe foods, you can move on to Phase III.

Phase II: Food intolerance self-test

During the four-week period of Phase II you will continue to eat only from the 'yes' list on page 173 and to avoid all the foods in the 'no' list – with one exception. One by one, under controlled conditions, you will also eat four previously prohibited foods to see whether or not they are problem foods for you and write any reactions in the Results column. These foods are suspected 'allergens' and will be tested at the rate of one per week as described below. This test only works when you have not consumed the foods in question for several weeks.

Testing procedure	Results
Week 1 **WHEAT TEST**	In addition to the 'yes' list, also consume egg-free wheat pasta, wheat flour or plain wheat crackers every day for five days, then stop. If you get any unpleasant reactions, such as headaches, sinus congestion or drowsiness, or if your weight rises by several pounds, make a note of these reactions and stop eating the wheat before the five days are up. There is no point in continuing, because it is likely that you have a wheat intolerance and need to continue avoiding wheat.	
	Whether or not you experience a reaction, stop the wheat after five days and eat only from the 'yes' list for the next two days. Do not eat any more wheat until the end of Phase II.	
Week 2 **DAIRY TEST**	Repeat what you did in Week 1, consuming cow's milk products daily instead of wheat, particularly fresh milk, cheese and yoghurt. The procedure is exactly the same as for Week 1. Do not eat any more cow's milk products until the end of Phase II.	
Week 3 **EGG TEST**	Repeat what you did in Week 1, consuming eggs daily instead of wheat. If you do not want to eat a whole egg every day, make a two-egg omelette with plain egg and water, cook it very thinly and eat a small strip each day for the test period. Do not eat any more egg until the end of Phase II.	
Week 4 **YEAST TEST**	Repeat what you did in Week 1, consuming yeast daily instead of wheat. Buy a small jar of low-sodium yeast extract from a health food store, and make it into a hot drink with boiling water. Drink this each day for the test period.	

CHAPTER 14

Phase III of the Waterfall Diet: Keeping water retention away

Phase III of the Waterfall Diet is designed for keeping water retention away and should be followed permanently. It is more relaxed and allows you a wide variety of foods. In fact, Phase III of the Waterfall Diet is less a diet and more a long-term eating strategy, encouraging you to be conscious of foods that aggravate or fight your specific type of water retention and to eat accordingly. It consists of the following three rules:

1. Continue to avoid any foods which tested as 'unsafe' during Phase II.
2. Continue eating as often as you can the special Waterfall Diet foods listed on page 176.
3. Follow the 90 per cent rule.

Unsafe foods

You should continue to avoid eating any 'unsafe' foods for at least six months. After six months, your body should have recovered enough for you to be able to eat your unsafe foods occasionally without causing a return of symptoms. But you will always need to be careful. I recommend that you save these foods for when you go out, as they are in any case difficult to avoid in restaurants, dinner parties and so on. Just try not to eat them at home.

You will need to continue reading food labels carefully. A lot of people fall by the wayside because they think 'a little bit' won't have any effect. Nothing could be further from the truth. If consumed regularly enough, just a teaspoon of one of your unsafe foods will take you right back to square one. Food intolerances have no mercy!

If it turned out that you have no unsafe foods and your water retention is not caused by a food intolerance, then your health needs more long-term work to reverse any metabolic imbalances which are causing your water retention. So Phase III is perhaps the most important stage of all.

Special Waterfall Diet foods

These foods help to correct the causes of your water retention and can also help to prevent these causes from returning. Blue, dark red and purple fruits and a little citrus peel and zest from time to time are very important. If you are a woman, don't forget to eat broccoli, cauliflower, cabbage or Brussels sprouts as often as you can. These help to prevent the high oestrogen levels which are linked not just with water retention, but with many female problems such as fibroids, ovarian cysts and breast cancer. Also important is the regular consumption of soya milk, tofu and iodine-rich foods such as sea fish and a little seaweed.

The 90 per cent rule

Starting with Phase III, the ban is partially lifted on foods such as tea and coffee, red meat, sugar and so on, which were on the 'no' list and were not included in the Phase II test. All these foods individually cause minor stress to your body. When you add them all up together and consume them regularly, this stress may no longer be so minor.

You do not have to avoid these foods completely, but think about consuming them once or twice a week instead of several times every day. Try not to slide back into old habits. If the amount of stress on your liver, your metabolism rises too much, your health may start to break down again, leading to the return of old symptoms and problems. I recommend that you restrict these foods to 10 per cent or less of your diet. It would be best if the remaining 90 per cent of your diet consists of foods from the Waterfall Diet 'yes' list on page 173.

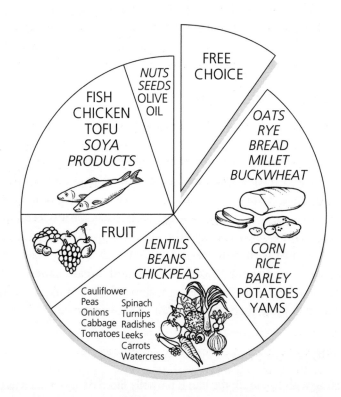

The rules of healthy eating: In Phase 3 of the Waterfall Diet, the foods you eat should match the proportions shown on the plate above. If you are a vegetarian, or if you do not eat fish or poultry regularly, you should ensure that you eat a selection every day of the vegetables, grains and other foods shown on the plate in italics.

> **Important note**
>
> If, after starting Phase III, you notice a return of any health problems such as joint pains, skin rashes or digestive problems, which had disappeared during Phase I, keep a diary of what you eat, what symptoms you experience and when you experience them. This will help you to identify what foods, such as occasional red meat, food additives and so on, might be responsible. If you are not able to identify the causes of your symptoms on your own, consider consulting a nutritional therapist (*see Useful Addresses on p.276*).

Dietary supplements (optional)

It is not essential to take dietary supplements with the Waterfall Diet. Many people believe that all of us get all the vitamins and minerals we need from a good, healthy diet, and this is true provided that you don't have extra needs due to absorption problems as we discussed on page 135. If you already eat a healthy diet but still have some of the signs of nutritional deficiencies listed below, then perhaps you are one of those people with extra high needs.

Symptoms and signs of various nutritional deficiencies

bad condition of skin or hair
birth defects in the newborn
bouts of depression unrelated to external events
deteriorating memory
easy exhaustion
eye and ear problems
heart (artery) disease
increasing mental confusion
infertility

kidney stones
menopausal symptoms
mental illness (in combination with extreme stress)
osteoporosis (brittle bone disease)
period pains
premenstrual syndrome
senility
sensitivity to chemicals
spasms
tendency to catch colds and flu easily
tendency to suffer from thrush/yeast infections
uncharacteristic mood swings and unusual aggression

When using dietary supplements, it is usually a good idea to take a multivitamin and multimineral preparation to use as a foundation. This helps to prevent imbalances caused by taking one nutrient on its own for too long. Check the labels so that the combination of products you take provides approximately the following:

Recommended basic multivitamin and mineral formula

vitamin A	7,500 iu[1]
vitamin B_1, B_2, B_6	25–50 mg
vitamin B_{12}	50 mcg
niacin (vitamin B_3)	50 mg
folic acid	400 mcg
pantothenic acid (vitamin B_5)	50 mg
vitamin C	100 mg
vitamin D	200 iu[2]
vitamin E	50 iu[3]

1. 1 iu = 0.3 micrograms (mcg or ug) of vitamin A
2. 1 iu = 0.025 micrograms of vitamin D
3. 1 iu = approx 1.5 milligrams (mg) of vitamin E.

boron	2 mg
chromium	50 mcg
copper	0.5 mg (500 mcg)
iron	5 mg
manganese	5 mg
selenium	50 mcg
zinc	10 mg
evening primrose, borage or blackcurrant seed oil[4]	250 mg
fish oil[5]	250 mg

Values given for minerals are elemental (i.e. for the mineral only, not for compounds such as magnesium oxide or chromium picolinate, which may contain only a small proportion of the mineral itself). Check your supplement labels to ensure that the manufacturer also gives elemental values.

Children: Reduce dosages in proportion to body weight.

Pregnancy: The above dosages are considered safe in pregnancy.

Magnesium (approx 100–200 mg/day) will normally need to be taken separately, since adding the required amount to a multinutrient formula would make each tablet or capsule too bulky. Many people also take additional vitamin C, up to 1,000 mg a day, to help combat pollution and prevent infections. If these amounts of vitamin C look very large to you, remember that almost all other mammals produce (proportionally) much more vitamin C than this in their own bodies every day. Humans are missing the last

4. The active nutritional ingredient in these oils is gamma linolenic acid (GLA).
5. The active nutritional ingredients in these oils are eicosapentaenoic acid (EPA) and docosahexaenoic acid (DHA). Fish oil supplements are not the same as fish liver oils, which contain little EPA and DHA but are a good source of vitamin A.

stage in the liver enzyme process which produces vitamin C from glucose.

For help with finding suitable nutritional or herbal supplements, sign up for my e-mail newsletters at my website (www.health-diets.net).

SECTION III

Waterfall Diet Recipes

CHAPTER 15

Delicious meals to make at home

These recipes are suitable for all phases of the Waterfall Diet, and particularly for Phase I.

Special Notes

If you don't eat chicken or fish please be sure to include rice (or rice cakes) and nuts or tofu in every meal. One meal a day must also include beans or lentils. Don't try to eat more sheep or goat's cheese or yoghurt instead – even non-cow dairy items are deliberately kept in low quantities on the Waterfall Diet.

You may find the first seven days a little monotonous, but please bear with the plan. Remember that the Waterfall Diet is a medical diet which aims to tackle the causes of water retention, so it will work better if certain items are consumed every day. If you want, you can vary the times you consume them. To improve the daily celery and radish juice, experiment with different flavours: try adding tomato, lemon or apple juice or a bit of chilli.

If you need a more substantial breakfast you can add any of the items listed under 'Snacks'. For instance corn thins or Scottish oatcakes with pure olive oil spread and sugar-free black cherry jam or crunchy peanut butter.

The Waterfall Diet is not calorie-controlled, but it is based on healthy eating principles. It is up to you to eat sensible portion sizes that do not leave you feeling hungry. If you eat slowly you will find that you are satisfied more easily.

Salt substitutes are products such as 'No Salt' (from Prewett) or 'Salt Rite' (in the UK) and 'Also Salt' or 'Morton Salt' (in the US). Please use them sparingly.

Recipes for the 7-day menu plan

Monday

Aduki bean salad with parsley, chopped celery and French dressing

Ingredients for 2 servings
   2 handfuls of home-cooked aduki beans or 1 can of aduki beans
      (in water)
   4 tbsp French dressing (*see recipe, p.268*)
   1 stick of celery
   2 tbsp fresh parsley, roughly chopped

The beans should be warm (ideally freshly cooked). Otherwise, drain them thoroughly and shake them around for a few minutes in a dry frying pan (skillet) over a medium heat until all moisture has evaporated and they are warmed through.

Transfer to a container and stir in the French dressing, followed by the remaining ingredients.

Broccoli soup with chives and parsley

Ingredients for 2–3 servings

- 1 medium head of broccoli or celery, or a small head of cauliflower, or 4 large handfuls of watercress or ½ lb (230 g) Brussels sprouts
- 1 large potato, chopped
- 1 large onion, chopped
- 34 fl oz/1 litre water
- 1 tbsp fresh parsley, chopped
- 1 tbsp fresh chives, snipped
- salt substitute
- ground black pepper to taste
- 3 tbsp soya cream

If using broccoli, peel the stalk first. Chop the vegetables into smallish pieces, then place in a lidded saucepan with the water, bring to the boil and simmer until tender (about 15 minutes). Remove from the heat. Liquidise the soup in the pan with a hand blender and finally stir in the parsley, chives, seasonings and soya cream.

(You can also use this recipe to make celery, cauliflower, watercress or Brussels sprout soup.)

Grilled or baked white fish with baked potato(es), braised vegetables and a sheep's yoghurt topping

Ingredients for each serving

   1 white fish fillet
   1 medium-to-large potato
   1 generous handful of chopped vegetables (e.g. carrots and cabbage)
   1 small onion, chopped
   1 tbsp fresh parsley, chopped
   salt substitute
   freshly ground black pepper
   olive oil
   2 tbsp sheep's yoghurt

Pre-heat the oven to 350°F/180°C/gas mark 4.

Prick the potato all over with a fork and bake in the oven for 45–60 minutes until soft.

Meanwhile put the chopped vegetables, onions, parsley and seasonings in a small saucepan with a tablespoon of olive oil and 2 tablespoons of water. Cover tightly and leave to braise over the lowest possible heat until tender (about 30 minutes). Check from time to time that the vegetables have not dried out and if necessary add another tablespoon of water from time to time.

Brush the fish with olive oil and place under the grill (broiler) for 2–5 minutes, depending on the thickness of the fish. Turn over and cook the other side until the fish flakes easily. Alternatively, after oiling the fish you can wrap it in foil and place on a baking tray in the oven to cook with the potato.

When ready, open the top of the potato, spoon the braised vegetables over it, followed by the sheep's yoghurt, and serve with the fish.

Stewed blueberries

For each serving you will need a generous handful of fresh or frozen blueberries.

If frozen, allow the fruits to defrost. Place the fruits in a small saucepan with two tablespoons of water. Warm the berries over a low heat, stirring from time to time, until they split and the juices run (approximately 20 minutes). Add a sprinkling of cinnamon and serve hot or cold.

Tuesday

Broad bean soup with parsley

Ingredients for 3–4 servings
    4 generous handfuls of fresh or frozen broad beans
    1 large potato, chopped
    34 fl oz/1 litre water
    2 tbsp fresh parsley, chopped
    salt substitute
    freshly ground black pepper

Fresh broad beans should be popped out of their skins before cooking.

Put the broad beans and chopped potato in a pan with the water and bring to the boil. Simmer for 15 minutes or until tender, then liquidise in the pan with a stick blender. Stir in the chopped parsley and seasonings before serving.

Tofu, mushroom and broccoli stir-fry with rice noodles

Ingredients for 2 servings
    8 oz/230 g firm tofu*
    1 tbsp rice flour
    salt substitute
    olive oil
    kettle of boiling water
    4 oz/115 g mushrooms, sliced
    florets from one medium-sized head of broccoli**
    1 clove garlic, chopped
    4 oz/115 g rice vermicelli***
    tamari sauce to taste
    pinch of chilli flakes

Drain the tofu and cut into bite-size cubes. Pat dry with absorbent kitchen paper. Sprinkle with rice flour and salt substitute and roll the cubes around in the flour to coat them lightly.

Heat 4 tbsp olive oil in a stir-fry pan over a high heat until it is hot enough to get a good sizzle when you add a tofu cube. Now add all the cubes, and fry until golden, turning them over after 1–2 minutes to cook the other side. When cooked, remove from the pan and put to one side.

Replace the pan on the heat, and add the mushrooms, plus a little more olive oil if necessary. Stir-fry them briskly for 1–2 minutes over a high heat, then remove and put to one side.

Replace the pan on the heat, add 4 tbsp water and the broccoli florets. Bring to the boil then cover the pan tightly, reduce the heat to the lowest possible setting and leave the broccoli to steam for 5

* The UK Cauldron brand is good for this, or Mori-Nu firm organic. Don't use silken tofu for this recipe as it is too soft.
** The broccoli stems can be saved for making broccoli juice or soup.
*** Brown rice vermicelli is best. This is sold as a brand from the Far East called X.O. and your local Asian shop may be able to order it for you. It is delicious and cooks very well.

minutes, checking that they do not dry out. Remove from the pan and put to one side.

Add 1 tbsp olive oil to the pan, followed by the garlic, and fry for 10 seconds. Remove from the heat.

Meanwhile, put the rice vermicelli in a bowl and cover generously with boiling water. Leave to soften for the length of time recommended on the packet, then drain into a sieve. Put the drained vermicelli into the stir-fry pan with the oil and garlic, add a few dashes of tamari sauce and the chilli flakes, place over a medium heat, and stir. Keep stirring the vermicelli until no more moisture is left in the pan, then add the cooked tofu cubes, mushrooms and broccoli. Stir together well, season, cover the pan, leave on a very low heat until all the ingredients are heated through, then serve.

Wednesday

Hummus

In this recipe a cup means an ordinary teacup.

Ingredients for 4 servings
　　1½ cups freshly cooked chick peas
　　½ cup cooking liquid from the chick peas
　　2 heaped tbsp sesame seeds
　　4 tbsp extra virgin olive oil
　　1 tbsp lemon juice
　　1 clove garlic, crushed
　　salt substitute
　　cayenne pepper to taste

Blend all the ingredients together in a food processor, adding more cooking liquid if necessary, until the mixture achieves the consistency of a thick dip. Use as a dip for crudités or rice or corn crackers. You could also slit open a flatbread (*see recipe, p.270*) and stuff with hummus mixed with alfalfa sprouts, green pepper strips and grated radish.

Watercress soup with chives and parsley

Ingredients for 3–4 servings
   1 medium onion, diced
   3 cups/150 g fresh watercress, chopped
   1 large potato, chopped
   34 fl oz/1 litre water
   1 tbsp soya cream
   1 tbsp fresh parsley, chopped
   1 tbsp fresh chives, chopped
   salt substitute
   freshly ground black pepper

Put the diced onion, chopped watercress and potato in a pan with the water and bring to the boil. Simmer for 15 minutes or until tender, then liquidise in the pan with a stick blender.

Stir in the soya cream, parsley, chives and seasoning before serving.

Gluten-free pasta bake with chicken strips and vegetables

Ingredients for 2–3 servings

8 oz/230 g fresh or frozen vegetables, chopped (e.g. carrots, cabbage, broccoli, spring greens, squash)

olive oil

water

2 cloves garlic, peeled and chopped

8 oz/230 g fresh organic chicken meat, cut into strips

1 rounded tbsp rice flour

34 fl oz/1 litre soya milk

8 oz/230 g pasta spirals made from rice or corn

freshly ground black pepper

salt substitute

Pre-heat the oven to 350°F/180°C/gas mark 4.

In a large saucepan, gently fry the chopped vegetables in a few tablespoons of olive oil until beginning to soften. Add a few tablespoons of water, cover the pan tightly and leave to braise over a low heat for 15 minutes or until just tender. Stir in the chopped garlic. Remove the pan from the heat.

Fry the chicken strips in a little olive oil over a medium heat for 5–10 minutes until browned all over. Remove from the pan and put to one side.

Add 2 tablespoons of olive oil to the same pan, sprinkle in the rice flour, and stir together thoroughly with a wooden spoon. Now add a little soya milk, stirring vigorously as you do so. When it starts to bubble, add a little more soya milk, always stirring. Keep adding the soya milk a little at a time until it is all in the pan. If any lumps have formed, use a hand blender to smooth them out. Continuing to stir, bring the pan up to the boil, then simmer gently until the sauce thickens. Simmer for a further 2 minutes then remove from the heat.

Meanwhile, cook the pasta spirals according to the directions on the packet until they are just *al dente*. (Do not overcook them as they will continue cooking in the oven.)

As soon as they are ready, run some cold water into the pan, drain them, return to the pan and combine the pasta with the cooked vegetables and chicken strips.

When the sauce is ready, stir it into the pasta, chicken and vegetable mix, season with salt substitute and freshly ground black pepper and transfer to an oven-proof dish. Cover the dish and bake in the oven for 45 minutes. Remove the cover for the last 10 minutes so that the top can brown a little.

Thursday

Hot mung bean soup with garlic, ginger and parsley

Ingredients for 3–4 servings

    17 fl oz/½ litre cooked, drained mung beans, measured in a
       measuring jug
    2 shallots, chopped
    2 tbsp olive oil
    1 clove garlic, chopped
    34 fl oz/1 litre water
    1 piece of fresh ginger the size of your thumb, peeled and
       chopped
    2 tbsp fresh parsley, chopped
    salt substitute
    freshly ground black pepper

To cook beans, see page 272.

Gently fry the chopped shallot in olive oil for a few minutes until softened. Add the chopped garlic and cook for a further 30 seconds before removing from the heat.

Put the mung beans in a pan with the water and ginger and bring to the boil. Simmer for a few minutes, then liquidise in the pan with a stick blender. Stir in the garlic, shallots, seasoning and parsley before serving.

Prawn Thai curry with broccoli

Ingredients for 2 servings
    10 fl oz/300 ml water
    1 inch/2½ cm piece cut from a block of creamed coconut
    2 tsp red Thai curry paste
    salt substitute
    florets from 1 medium-sized head of broccoli (the broccoli
        stems can be saved for making broccoli juice or soup).
    2 generous handfuls of fresh or frozen prawns (shrimps)

Put the water, creamed coconut, curry paste and seasoning into a saucepan and bring to the boil, stirring until everything is dissolved. Add the broccoli florets and simmer gently for 5 minutes. Add the prawns, wait for the water to come back to simmering point and simmer gently for a further 30 seconds. Serve with brown rice (*see p.272*).

Friday

Rainbow salad

Ingredients for 2 servings
   4 inch/10 cm piece of white mooli or icicle radish
   1 large carrot
   1 small beetroot (beet), raw or cooked
   1 medium yellow pepper (bell pepper)
   lettuce leaves, shredded
   4 tbsp French dressing (*see recipe, p.268*)

Using a food processor, finely grate the radish, followed by the carrot and beetroot, in that order. Keep separate to avoid staining. If you don't have a food processor, then use a coarse hand grater instead.

Cut the yellow pepper into long, thin strips.

Now layer the vegetables, putting the lettuce leaves at the bottom, followed by a layer of beetroot, then yellow pepper, then a layer of radish and finally a layer of carrot.

Just before serving, pour the dressing over the top.

Hot aduki bean soup with miso, ginger, parsley and arame

Ingredients for 3–4 servings

>   17 fl oz/½ litre cooked, drained aduki beans, measured in a
>   measuring jug
>   2 shallots, chopped
>   2 tbsp olive oil
>   1 tbsp wheat-free miso
>   34 fl oz/1 litre water
>   1 piece of fresh ginger the size of your thumb, peeled and
>   chopped
>   1 small handful arame seaweed
>   salt substitute
>   freshly ground black pepper
>   2 tbsp fresh parsley, chopped

To cook beans, see page 272.

Gently fry the chopped shallots in olive oil for a few minutes until softened. Remove from the heat.

Put the aduki beans in a pan with the miso, water and ginger, and bring to the boil. Stir well to dissolve the miso. Simmer for a few minutes, then liquidise in the pan with a stick blender. Stir in the arame, shallots, seasoning and parsley. Stand for a few minutes to allow the arame to soften before serving.

Baked salmon parcels with new potatoes and cucumber salad

Ingredients for 2 servings
    new potatoes (enough for two servings)
    2 salmon fillets weighing about 4 oz/115 g each
    olive oil
    salt substitute
    freshly ground black pepper
    fresh dill, roughly chopped
    1 lime, thinly sliced
    ½ cucumber
    2 tbsp French dressing (*see recipe, p.268*) or soya yoghurt
        (*see recipe, p.269*)

Put the new potatoes into a steamer and cook until tender (20–30 minutes).

Pre-heat the oven to 350°F/180°C/gas mark 4.

Brush the salmon fillets with olive oil then season with salt substitute and freshly ground black pepper. Sprinkle a pinch of chopped dill over the fish, then lay 3 overlapping slices of lime on top.

Place each fillet carefully in the centre of a piece of baking foil and fold the foil around the fish, tucking in the edges to make a parcel. If you wish to avoid aluminium, it is possible to make the parcels with baking parchment or grease-proof paper instead, in which case use a stapler to hold the edges of the parcel together.

Lay the parcels in an open oven-proof dish or tray and bake in the oven for 25 minutes or until the fish is opaque throughout. Never overcook fish – it is at its best when only just done.

Meanwhile, dice the cucumber, place in a bowl, dress with French dressing or soya yoghurt and sprinkle with chopped dill.

When the fish is ready, serve immediately with the new potatoes and cucumber salad.

Exotic warm fruit salad in grape juice

Ingredients for 4 servings
  1 peach, thinly sliced
  1 small mango, skinned and chopped
  1 kiwi fruit, peeled and sliced
  2 slices fresh pineapple (or canned pineapple in juice, drained)
  2 tbsp fresh or frozen (defrosted) blueberries
  2 tbsp red grape juice

Pre-heat the oven to 350°F/180°C/gas mark 4.

Place the fruits in an oven-proof dish, pour the grape juice over them and cover with a well-fitting lid. Cook in the oven for 15–20 minutes then serve immediately.

Saturday

Fried herring cakes with mushrooms and grilled tomatoes

Ingredients for 2 servings
   2 medium herrings, scaled, trimmed and gutted
   2 dessertspoons chickpea (gram) flour
   salt substitute
   freshly ground black pepper
   olive oil
   4 large open mushrooms
   2 large tomatoes, cut in half

Poach the herrings in a few tablespoons of water in a lidded pan over a low heat for 10 minutes, until the fish comes apart easily. Allow the fish to cool, then slit it open lengthwise and carefully remove all the bones.

Using a fork, mash the fish with the chickpea flour and seasonings, then, using your hands, divide it into four balls and form each ball into a fairly thin patty. Dust the outside of the patties with more chickpea flour.

Heat 2 tbsp olive oil in a frying pan (skillet) over a fairly high heat, then put the patties into the pan and fry for 1–2 minutes on each side or until brown. Keep them warm until the mushrooms and tomatoes are ready.

Brush the mushrooms and tomatoes liberally with olive oil and season them. Lay them face up on a heat-proof dish under a hot grill (broiler) and cook for 2–3 minutes until the mushrooms are juicy and the tomatoes beginning to brown. Serve immediately.

The herring cakes can be prepared the night before for cooking in the morning.

Soya milk, banana and purple fruit smoothie

Ingredients for 2 servings
   17 fl oz / ½ litre soya milk
   1 banana
   1 handful fresh or frozen blueberries or black forest fruits

Add all the ingredients to a blender or smoothie-maker and whizz until smooth. Drink immediately.

Note: This recipe will instead produce a soft ice cream if you add frozen fruit and frozen banana pieces to the soya milk before blending. In this case, use a food processor instead of a blender.

Red Thai curry with chicken, vegetables and rice noodles

Ingredients for 2 servings

  olive oil
  8 oz/230 g raw organic chicken meat, cut into bite-size pieces
  2 tsp red Thai curry paste (more if you like it hotter)
  8 oz/230 g fresh or frozen vegetables, chopped (e.g. carrots,
      cabbage, broccoli, spring greens, squash)
  1 can of coconut milk
  4 oz/115 g rice vermicelli*
  kettle of boiling water
  salt substitute

Heat 4 tbsp olive oil in a large saucepan over a high heat until it is hot enough to get a good sizzle when you add a piece of chicken.

Now add all the chicken pieces and fry until golden, turning them over after 1–2 minutes to cook the other side. When cooked, add the curry paste and stir to incorporate. Now add the vegetables and coconut milk. Bring up to simmering point, put the lid on the pan and simmer gently until the vegetables are tender and the chicken cooked through (15–20 minutes).

Meanwhile, put the rice vermicelli in a bowl and cover generously with boiling water. Leave to soften for the length of time recommended on the packet, then drain into a sieve. Put the drained vermicelli with 2 tbsp olive oil into a stir-fry pan, place over a medium heat, and stir. Keep stirring the vermicelli until no more moisture is left in the pan, then transfer to a serving dish. Pour the chicken and vegetable curry over the top.

---

* Brown rice vermicelli is best. This is sold as a brand from the Far East called X.O. and your local Asian shop may be able to order it for you. It is delicious and cooks very well.

Brown rice pudding made with soya milk and cinnamon and topped with sugar-free black cherry jam

Ingredients for 4 servings

4 oz/115 g short grain brown rice which has been soaked
   overnight in water and then drained

34 fl oz/1 litre carton soya milk

1 date (stoned)

1 pinch cinnamon

sugar-free black cherry jam (e.g. St Dalfour brand sweetened
   with fruit juice instead of sugar)

Place the rice, soya milk, date and cinnamon in a heavy-bottomed saucepan (enamelled cast iron is best) and bring to a gentle simmer, stirring from time to time. Put a heat diffuser under the pan and leave on the lowest setting with the lid on tightly for 1 hour. Check occasionally to ensure that the rice pudding is not beginning to stick to the bottom of the pan, and stir gently. The date acts to sweeten the rice pudding and should dissolve completely during the cooking process.

When ready, serve each portion topped with a teaspoon of sugar-free black cherry jam.

Sunday

Kedgeree

Ingredients for 1 serving

4 oz / 115 g cod, haddock or salmon fillet, skinned
2 tbsp water
2 tbsp extra virgin olive oil
4 tbsp small frozen peas
Few drops Tabasco sauce
1 tsp tamari sauce
1 portion cooked brown rice
1 tbsp mushroom pieces which have been quickly fried in olive oil
1 tsp fresh parsley, chopped

Place the fish in a pan with enough water to come halfway up the fish. Bring to simmering point then put the lid on and simmer very gently for 5 minutes, or until the fish flakes easily. Meanwhile, heat the olive oil in a heavy-bottomed saucepan, or preferably a stir-fry pan, and add the frozen peas. Stir-fry over a medium heat until they have defrosted and any water has evaporated. Then add the Tabasco sauce and tamari sauce, followed by the rice and mushrooms and stir in with the peas. Turn down the heat to very low, sprinkle in the water and cover with a lid or plate.

While the rice is heating, drain the fish and separate into flakes.

When the rice has heated through, remove from the heat and add the fish flakes, folding them into the rice very gently so that they do not break.

Serve sprinkled with fresh chopped parsley.

Variations
For a more risotto-like texture, you could stir in some warm soya cream before adding the fish.

Soya milk, avocado and banana smoothie

Ingredients for 3–4 servings
  34 fl oz /1 litre soya milk
  1 banana
  1 avocado pear

Add all the ingredients to a blender or smoothie-maker and whizz until smooth. Drink immediately.

Potato pancake with goat's cheese and spinach

Ingredients for 1 serving
  2 tbsp olive oil
  2 medium-sized waxy potatoes
  salt substitute
  freshly ground black pepper
  2 oz /55g fresh young spinach, washed and shredded
  2 oz /55g soft goat's cheese, cut into pieces

Pre-heat a 9½ inch /25 cm diameter frying-pan (skillet) over a medium heat until very hot, then add the olive oil. Coarsely grate the potatoes as quickly as you can to prevent browning, then transfer them to the hot frying pan. Using the tip of a spatula, distribute them evenly in the pan and press down to flatten. Cover the frying pan and leave the pancake to cook for 1 minute.

Turn the heat down low-to-medium, season the top of the pancake and leave it to cook for a further 9 minutes with the lid on the pan. Check from time to time that the pancake is still sizzling underneath but not getting too dark brown.

Remove the pan from the heat and carefully slide the pancake on to a large plate. Replace the pan over a medium heat and add another tablespoon of oil. Cover the pancake with a second plate, then invert the plates, thus turning the pancake over. When the pan is sizzling hot again, carefully slide the pancake back into the pan to cook the other side and replace the lid. Turn the heat down again after 1 minute and then cook for a further 5 minutes. Remove from the pan and keep warm.

While the pancake is cooking, stir-fry the spinach in 2 tbsp hot olive oil until wilted. Remove from the heat and spoon on to one half of the potato pancake. Cover with the pieces of soft goat's cheese, season, then fold the other half of the pancake over the filling and serve.

Black forest gelled fruits with soya cream

Ingredients for each serving

1 portion of hot fruit compote (*see recipe, p.259*)
gelatine or vegetarian gelling agent

Using the directions on the packet of gelatine or vegetarian gelling agent, calculate how much you will need and prepare it as directed.

Add the gelling agent to the hot fruit compote and stir to incorporate. Leave to cool and set before serving with soya cream.

More recipes

The following recipes are for use after the first seven days of Phase I but if necessary can also be used to provide substitutes during the first seven days.

Breakfast

Sheep's milk or soya yoghurt with almonds and apple compote

Ingredients for 1 serving
Swirl 4 tbsp sheep's milk or soya yoghurt (*see recipe, p.269*) into a generous serving of apple compote (*see fruit compote recipe on p.259*). Sprinkle liberally with toasted flaked almonds.

Sultana and sunflower seed porridge with soya milk and soya cream

Ingredients for 1 serving
- 3 dessertspoons porridge oats or medium-ground oatmeal
- 1 mug unsweetened soya milk
- 2 tsp sultanas
- 2 tsp sunflower seeds
- soya cream to serve

Put the porridge oats or medium-ground oatmeal and 1 mug of unsweetened soya milk in a small, heavy-bottomed saucepan (enamelled cast iron if you have one). Bring to the boil, stirring constantly, then turn down the heat to a simmer and add the sultanas and sunflower seeds. Keep stirring for a minute or two until it thickens. Add a little more soya milk when ready if you prefer a more runny porridge. Serve with a little soya cream poured over the top.

Variation
Soak the sultanas and sunflower seeds in the soya milk overnight before making the porridge.

Authentic Swiss muesli with flaked nuts and sweet apricots

Ingredients for 1 serving
   3 tbsp medium or fine-ground oatmeal
   water
   soya or nut milk to taste
   1 unsulphured* dried apricot, chopped small
   1 tbsp flaked nuts

Did you know that the Swiss never eat muesli straight out of the packet? They know that raw grains should always be soaked overnight before eating them, because this breaks down mildly poisonous chemicals they contain, known as enzyme inhibitors, that can upset your intestines.

Soak the oatmeal overnight in the water. The amount of water you need will depend on how much the oatmeal can absorb – about three times its volume for medium oatmeal, and more for fine oatmeal. If you find after an hour or so that the mixture has become too solid, add more water. No milk is necessary since the oats create their own milk. In the morning, check the consistency and add a little soya or nut milk if you wish, to achieve your pre-ferred consistency. If you use fine oatmeal, the result will be very creamy. Stir in the dried apricot pieces and sprinkle with flaked nuts.

---

* Dried apricots are orange in colour if treated with sulphur dioxide. This additive is an intestinal irritant and can cause bloating and gas. Unsulphured apricots (from health food stores) are dark brown and much sweeter in flavour.

Soups and salads

Lentil soup with miso, celery and onion

Ingredients for 6 servings
- ½ pint/275 ml dried brown, red or puy lentils
- 1 large onion, chopped
- 6 sticks celery, chopped
- 34 fl oz/1 litre water
- 1 heaped tbsp wheat-free miso paste
- 1 tbsp unsalted tomato purée (optional)
- ¼ tsp mixed dried herbs
- pinch cayenne pepper

Simmer the ingredients together until cooked (about 30 minutes). Thicken by partially liquidising with a hand blender.

Shredded white cabbage with grated carrot in yoghurt and mustard vinaigrette

Ingredients for 1 serving

1 large handful finely shredded raw white cabbage
1 handful coarsely grated raw carrot
1 tbsp dry roasted unsalted peanuts, crushed (optional)
2 tbsp extra virgin olive oil
1 tsp lemon juice
½ tsp French mustard
1 tbsp soya yoghurt (*see recipe, p.269*)
salt substitute
ground black pepper to taste

Combine the shredded cabbage and carrot in a bowl, plus the peanuts if you are using them. Whip the oil, lemon juice, French mustard, soya yoghurt and seasonings together in a small dish and pour over the vegetable mixture.

Broccoli in vinaigrette with sliced spring onion

Ingredients for 3 servings

1 spring onion (scallion), finely sliced
French dressing to taste (*see recipe, p.268*)
1 medium head of broccoli

Mix the sliced spring onion with the French dressing. Cut the head off the broccoli stem. Peel the stem (or save it for juicing) and separate the head into small florets. Steam the florets for 12–15 minutes or until just tender. Pour over the French dressing and spring onion mixture and gently turn the florets until the dressing is evenly distributed.

Can be eaten warm or cold. Try it served on a bed of alfalfa sprouts.

Tomato slices on a bed of alfalfa sprouts and grated radish with French dressing and tofu mayonnaise

Ingredients for 1 serving
- 1 large handful alfalfa sprouts
- 1 large handful grated mooli radish
- 1 beef tomato, sliced
- 3 tbsp French dressing (*see recipe, p.268*)
- 1 tbsp tofu mayonnaise (*see recipe, p.268*)

Place the alfalfa sprouts in a dish or lunch box, cover with grated radish and tomato slices, pour over French dressing then top with a dollop of tofu mayonnaise.

Beetroot and orange salad

Ingredients for 2 generous servings

- 1 raw beetroot, peeled and grated, or 1 cooked beetroot, chopped
- ½ orange lightly peeled, sliced
- ½ eating apple, chopped
- 8 black grapes, halved with seeds removed
- 1 stick celery, chopped
- 1 spring onion (scallion), sliced
- 6–8 freshly shelled walnuts chopped into fairly large pieces
- 4–6 sprigs watercress, roughly chopped

Dressing

- juice ½ orange (about 2 tbsp)
- 1 dessertspoon olive oil
- 1 tsp finely grated orange zest
- generous pinch mixed dried herbs
- salt substitute
- freshly ground black pepper

Prepare the dressing by mixing the orange juice with the olive oil and then whisking with a fork. Add the zest, herbs and black pepper. Prepare the fruit and vegetables and place in a salad dish. Pour the dressing over and serve immediately.

Main dishes

Spicy bean and vegetable rosti

Ingredients for 2 servings

9 oz/255 g cooked borlotti beans or black-eyed beans
½ small onion, finely chopped or grated
1 stick celery, finely chopped
1 tbsp unsalted tomato purée
2 rounded tsp dried parsley
½ tsp curry powder
salt substitute
ground black pepper
3 medium-sized potatoes
extra virgin olive oil for cooking

Mash the beans roughly with a fork, and mix with the remaining ingredients except the olive oil and potato. Form the bean mixture into 6 patties. Peel and grate the potato and squeeze out the excess water with your hands. Cover both sides of each bean pattie with grated potato and press gently between both hands. The potato will create quite a ragged covering, but this will adhere to the mixture when you start to cook the patties.

Gently heat a little olive oil in a heavy-bottomed frying pan. Slide a spatula under each rosti to transfer it to the pan and cook gently in batches of 2 or 3 for 5–8 minutes each side or until the potato is brown and crisp. Serve immediately with a mixed salad and a spoonful of soya yoghurt garnished with chopped coriander leaves.

Vegetable and lentil pasties

Ingredients to make 2 large pasties

1 small onion, finely chopped
extra virgin olive oil
2 oz/55 g shredded cabbage
2 oz/55 g frozen peas
2 oz/55 g cooked puy lentils (small green lentils)
1 tbsp unsalted tomato purée
1 dessertspoon soya yoghurt
½ tsp dried oregano
generous pinch mixed dried herbs
freshly grated nutmeg
salt substitute
ground black pepper
1 quantity of spelt pastry (*see recipe, p.270*)
1 tsp soya flour
4 tsp water
sesame seeds

Pre-heat the oven to 400°F/200°C/gas mark 6.

Gently cook the onions in a little olive oil until beginning to brown. Add cabbage, peas and lentils. Cook for 2–3 minutes. Add tomato purée, soya yoghurt, herbs, nutmeg, salt substitute and pepper. Set to one side.

Divide the pastry dough into 2 pieces. Roll out on a floured board, place a tea plate over the top and trim round with a knife so that you have a perfect round of dough. Brush a little cold water around the edge of the circle of pastry. Place some of the filling in the middle and fold in half to create a semi-circle. Seal the edges by pressing with a fork or the tip of a knife. Make 2 small incisions with a knife in the top of the pasty to allow steam to escape. Repeat until you have used all the ingredients.

To make a glaze, mix 1 tsp soya flour with 4 tsp water. Brush on to each pasty and sprinkle with sesame seeds.

Place the pasties on an oiled baking tray and bake for approximately 20–25 minutes or until golden brown.

Twice-baked potatoes

Ingredients for 2 servings
   2 baking potatoes, well scrubbed
   2 tbsp hummus (*see recipe, p.229*)
   1 tbsp finely chopped onion
   1 spring onion, finely sliced
   1 stick celery, finely chopped

Pre-heat the oven to 400°F/200°C/gas mark 6. Bake the potatoes until they feel soft when you squeeze them. Remove from oven and slice in half lengthways.

Scoop out the potato flesh, leaving the skins intact. Combine the potato, hummus, chopped onion, spring onion and celery, mixing well, and then pile into the potato skin halves. Place on an ovenproof dish and return to the oven. Bake for another 20 minutes or until the potato mixture is beginning to brown. Serve with the beetroot and orange salad (*see recipe, p.251*).

Red Thai curry with pan-fried tofu

Ingredients for 1 serving

3 thick slices from a block of firm tofu
salt substitute
cayenne pepper
groundnut oil for frying
¼ pint/150 ml water
2 tsp red Thai curry paste (more if you like it stronger)
½ inch/1 cm piece cut from a block of creamed coconut
½ cup mixed frozen vegetables (e.g. carrots and red sweet
    peppers diced small, peas, sweetcorn)
1 portion uncooked vermicelli rice noodles or 1 portion cooked
    brown rice

Cut the tofu into bite-size pieces, pat dry with kitchen paper and
sprinkle with salt substitute and cayenne pepper. Heat the groundnut oil to a depth of ¼ inch/½ cm in a frying pan. When hot
enough for the tofu to sizzle when added, carefully put the pieces
in the pan and fry on each side for 1–2 minutes or until golden.
Drain on kitchen paper.

Heat the water in a saucepan. Add the curry paste and creamed
coconut, stirring until dissolved. Add the frozen vegetables, put
the lid on the saucepan and simmer for a few minutes.

Place the vermicelli rice noodles in a bowl. Boil a kettleful of
water and pour the water generously over the noodles, leaving
them plenty of room to swell. Leave for 4 minutes then run a little
cold water into the bowl before draining the noodles thoroughly
in a large sieve. If using rice, heat the rice in a tightly lidded pan
over a low heat with a tablespoon of water.

When the vegetables are heated through, stir in the fried tofu
pieces and coat with the sauce. Serve the rice or noodles with the
vegetables and tofu on top and a little of the sauce spooned over.

Hawaiian tofu kebabs

Ingredients to serve 2

- 1 stick celery, cut into 8 x 1 inch/2½ cm pieces
- ½ red pepper, cut into 8 pieces
- ½ yellow or orange pepper, cut into 8 pieces
- 8 cherry tomatoes
- 8 button mushrooms
- 8 chunks of either fresh pineapple, or canned pineapple in juice (*not* syrup)
- 1 packet firm tofu, cut into 16 cubes
- sesame seeds

Marinade

- ½ tsp wheat-free miso
- 3 fl oz/75 ml pineapple juice, either extracted from fresh pineapple, or taken from the can
- 2 tbsp fresh orange juice
- 1 small clove garlic, crushed
- 1 pinch ground ginger
- ½ dessertspoon olive oil
- 2–3 drops tamari sauce
- freshly ground black pepper

Prepare the vegetables, pineapple and tofu and set aside.

To make the marinade, dissolve the miso paste in a little of the pineapple juice then combine with the remaining marinade ingredients in a large bowl.

Place the vegetables, pineapple and tofu in a large, shallow dish. Pour the marinade over and store in the fridge for at least one hour. Stir gently from time to time and spoon the marinade over the vegetables, making sure they're all well covered.

Thread the vegetables, pineapple and tofu chunks on to metal skewers. Pour the marinade into a saucepan and heat over a medium hob until reduced down and slightly thickened. Balance the threaded skewers over a shallow dish and either brush the thickened marinade on to each piece or drizzle over with a spoon. Sprinkle with sesame seeds if liked, and cook the kebabs under a pre-heated medium grill until the vegetables are tender and beginning to brown. Turn the skewers regularly to ensure the kebabs are browned on each side.

Serve the kebabs on a bed of long grain brown rice (*see page 272*), with a mixed salad and a side dish of soya yoghurt (*see recipe, p.269*) combined with finely chopped cucumber and fresh mint.

Nutty mushroom bake

In this recipe a cup is an ordinary teacup.

Ingredients for 3–4 servings

    1 onion, quartered
    2 sticks celery, roughly cut into segments
    1 small green pepper, cut into 8 pieces
    4 tbsp olive oil
    1 medium carrot, grated
    ¼ lb/115 g mushrooms, diced
    2 oz/55 g walnuts coarsely ground in food processor
    a few leaves of fresh basil, chopped, or ½ tsp dried basil
    ground black pepper
    tamari sauce
    2 cups cooked brown rice

Pre-heat the oven to 400°F/200°C/gas mark 6.

Grease a loaf tin.

Process the onion, celery and green pepper together in a food processor until finely chopped. Place a large, heavy-bottomed saucepan, or preferably a stir-fry pan, over a medium-high heat, and when hot, add 2 tbsp olive oil, followed by the onion, celery and green pepper mixture and the grated carrot. Stir-fry for 5 minutes until the mixture begins to soften, then take off the heat and transfer the contents to a bowl.

Clean and dry the pan then replace over a medium-high heat and add the chopped mushrooms. Stir-fry without oil for a minute to dry them out a little, then add the oil and continue to stir-fry until golden brown.

Take off the heat, replace the vegetables in the pan and mix in the chopped walnuts, basil, pepper and a few dashes of tamari sauce.

Finally, fold the rice in gently, ensuring that it does not break up.

Transfer the contents to a loaf tin, smooth down evenly with a fork, cover with foil and bake for about 40 minutes.

Serve with tomato slices on a bed of alfalfa sprouts and grated radish, with French dressing and tofu mayonnaise (*see recipes, p.268*).

Variations
Use cooked buckwheat or millet instead of brown rice, or include a tablespoon of wild rice.

Dessert recipes

Fresh fruit compote

Ingredients for each serving
> fresh or frozen sweet fruit: berries, cherries, apricots, peaches,
>   apples
> handful of raisins (if using apples)
> white grape juice, apple juice or orange juice (optional)

Some fruits may need the addition of a little grape or orange juice to make the compote juicy enough. If using apples, select a naturally sweet variety.

Cut the apples into quarters and remove the core, then cut into small pieces or slices, placing the pieces in a bowl of cold water until ready for cooking. Mix with a handful of raisins and a little apple juice or white grape juice before placing in the casserole dish and cooking (grape juice is the sweetest). If using frozen fruits, allow them to defrost first.

Place the fruit in an oven-proof casserole dish in a medium oven for 25 minutes or until the fruits split and the juices run. Serve warm or cold, with soya yoghurt (*see recipe, p.269*) or soya cream.

In Phase III of the diet, if you are allowed alcohol you can add some sweet red wine to the compote before cooking.

Date and chestnut dream

Ingredients for 1 serving

    4–5 unsweetened canned chestnuts (or boil fresh chestnuts until
       soft and shell them yourself)

    1 rounded tbsp date purée (*see recipe, p.269*)

    up to ¼ pint/150 ml soya cream

For the topping

    grated bitter chocolate

    1 black cherry

Mash the chestnuts using a fork, then mix with the date purée and most of the soya cream. Whizz with a blender until the mixture has the consistency of thick cream.

Serve in glass dishes with the remaining soya cream poured on top and decorate with a little grated bitter chocolate and a black cherry.

Chocolate banana cream boats

Ingredients for 6 servings

9 oz/250 g pack firm organic silken tofu

8 bananas, peeled

2 tsp cocoa powder

2 handfuls sunflower seeds

a few tablespoons of soya milk

pieces of fruit (canned mandarin orange segments, cherries, or
  chopped peach) or a sprig of mint and flaked nuts to garnish

Roughly chop the tofu and two of the bananas, then whizz in a
blender with the cocoa powder, sunflower seeds and some of the
soya milk until the mixture looks creamy. Add a little more soya
milk if the cream is too thick.

Cut the remaining 6 bananas lengthwise into halves and place
in pairs on a serving dish. Dollop each pair with the chocolate
banana cream and slightly press together to make a 'boat' shape.
Decorate with your chosen garnish and serve immediately.

You could also use the chocolate banana cream as a topping for
the blinis in the next recipe.

Black Forest blinis

Ingredients for approximately 16 blinis

For the blinis

4 oz/115 g buckwheat flour

1 oz/28 g soya flour

2 tsp ground cinnamon

1 tsp low-sodium baking powder

2 tbsp raisins

8 fl oz/225 ml soya milk

2 tbsp soya yoghurt *(see recipe, p.269)*

olive oil for cooking

For the topping
  sugar-free black cherry jam
  soya yoghurt (*see recipe, p.269*)
  a little grated bitter chocolate

To make the blinis, mix together the dry ingredients and raisins. Slowly add the soya milk to make a thick, pourable batter. Stir in the soya yoghurt and beat well with a wooden spoon. If necessary, add more liquid to achieve the right consistency, which should be similar to the batter used for 'drop scones': a spoonful dropped in the pan should spread out by itself to a thickness of about ¼ inch (½ cm).

Heat a heavy-bottomed frying pan on medium heat and wipe over with a wad of kitchen paper dipped in a little olive oil. Drop tablespoonfuls of the mixture into the hot pan and cook until small holes appear in the batter. Flip over, using a metal spatula, and cook the second side for about the same length of time. Re-oil the pan between each batch.

The blinis should be light, fluffy and slightly golden brown on the outside.

Serve warm, spread with the black cherry jam and a teaspoon of soya yoghurt. Sprinkle with the grated bitter chocolate.

Topping variations
A teaspoon of soya yoghurt sprinkled with toasted sesame seeds and topped with sliced fresh pear.
A teaspoon of banana cream (*see previous recipe*).
Apple and raisin compote or sugar-free marmalade plus a dollop of soya yoghurt.

Sultana and coconut cheesecakes

Ingredients to make 3 ramekins
  1 oz/28 g sultanas
  a few tablespoons of water
  ½ oz/15 g chopped mixed nuts
  ½ oz/15 g oatflakes
  ½ oz/15 g dessicated coconut
  ½ oz/15 g gelatine
  juice of 1 orange
  1 tsp natural vanilla extract
  9 oz/250 g pack firm organic silken tofu

Put the sultanas in a small saucepan with 4 tablespoons of water. Bring to the boil and simmer very gently for 10 minutes, adding a little more water if necessary to prevent them from boiling dry.

Meanwhile, lightly oil the inside of three ramekins or small moulds (about 3½ inches/9 cm) in diameter. Toast the chopped mixed nuts and oatflakes in a frying pan over a medium heat for 5 minutes until beginning to brown. Take off the heat and stir in the dessicated coconut. Divide this mixture between the ramekins and press down firmly.

Remove the sultanas from the heat. Sprinkle the gelatine on to 4 tablespoons of cold water in a heat-proof bowl or double-boiler and mix thoroughly, ensuring there are no lumps.

Once the mixture has turned into a thick paste, place the dish in or over a pan of boiling water. Stir the gelatine as it dissolves.

When fully dissolved, stir in the sultanas, orange juice and vanilla extract.

Using a hand blender, whizz this mixture into the tofu until smooth and creamy, then spoon into the ramekin dishes. Chill until set.

To turn out, stand the ramekin dishes in hot water for a minute, then turn upside-down.

Snack recipes

Carolyn's special spicy carrot cake

In this recipe a cup means an ordinary teacup.

Ingredients

 1 cup dates (stoned)
 1¼ cups water
 ¾ cup raisins
 2 large carrots, finely grated
 2 tsp mixed spice
 1¾ cups spelt flour
 ¼ cup soya flour
 2 tsp low-sodium baking powder
 1 cup chopped hazelnuts

Simmer the dates, water, raisins, carrots and mixed spice for 5 minutes. Cover and allow to stand overnight.

Pre-heat the oven to 325°F/170°C/gas mark 3.

Oil a 6–7 inch (15–18 cm) cake tin and line with greaseproof paper.

Combine the flours and baking powder and add them and the hazelnuts to the carrot mixture, mixing well. Bake for 1½–2 hours in the centre of the oven.

The cake is ready when a skewer comes out clean.

Derbyshire oatcakes

These delicious pancake-like oatcakes are usually made with a yeast batter, but this recipe, using a yoghurt-based mixture, is just as good and produces a lovely nutty texture. They can be eaten with savoury or sweet accompaniments or just on their own, as an alternative to bread or crackers.

Ingredients to make 6 oatcakes
 4 oz/115 g medium oatmeal
 4 oz/115 g spelt flour
 5 fl oz/150 ml soya milk (tepid)
 ½ pint/275 ml water (tepid)
 2 tbsp soya yoghurt (*see recipe, p.269*)
 2 tsp low-sodium baking powder

Mix the oatmeal and flour together in a large mixing bowl. Gradually stir in the soya milk, water and soya yoghurt using a large wooden spoon, then beat well until a smooth, thick batter is produced. Leave covered for 1 hour (or overnight if you will be eating the oatcakes for breakfast). Just before cooking, stir in the baking powder.

Heat a large, heavy-bottomed frying pan. Using a wad of kitchen paper dipped into a little olive oil, lightly wipe the surface of the hot pan. Using a ladle or small cup, pour about one-third of the batter into the pan. Immediately tilt and turn the pan so that the batter runs to the edge of the pan, forming a pancake shape. Cook the oatcake on a medium heat for about a minute or until it will leave the pan cleanly and is beginning to brown. Slide a metal spatula underneath and flip it over. Cook the second side for about the same time and stack the cooked oatcakes on a plate. Stir the batter regularly to keep the pouring consistency. Re-oil the pan between each batch.

If the oatcakes are not for eating immediately, stack them on a plate, separated by a layer of absorbent kitchen paper, as you cook them. Once cool, they will keep for a few days in the fridge and need only be briefly heated under the grill before eating. If freezing the oatcakes, first place them in the freezer individually, i.e. not in a stack, otherwise they will stick together as they freeze. They can be toasted straight from the freezer.

Roasted vegetable pissaladière

Ingredients for 1 serving
   extra virgin olive oil
   ½ yellow pepper, cut into chunks
   1 fresh ripe tomato, quartered
   5–6 button mushrooms, sliced
   1 small onion, thinly sliced
   1 round of flatbread dough, uncooked (*see recipe, p.270*)
   tomato purée
   6 black olives (choose a low-salt variety), pitted and halved
   mixed herbs
   freshly ground black pepper

Pre-heat the oven to 200°C/400°F/gas mark 6. Rub a little olive oil on to a roasting tray. Place the prepared vegetables on the tray and drizzle a few drops of olive oil over them. Roast for about 10 minutes or until the vegetables are beginning to soften and brown.

Oil a small, shallow oven-proof dish and place the dough round in the base. Spread a little tomato purée on the dough and pile the roasted vegetables on top. Garnish with the black olive halves and dot a little more tomato purée around the vegetables. Sprinkle with mixed herbs and a little black pepper. Bake for about 15–20 minutes. Check that the dough base is cooked through and then serve immediately.

Fruity almond cookies

So sweet, no one will realise they're made without sugar.

Ingredients to make 20 cookies
  4 oz/115 g unsulphured dried apricots
  water as required
  4 oz/115 g ground almonds
  2 oz/55 g chopped mixed nuts
  2 oz/55 g mixed dried fruit with peel
  2 oz/55 g soya flour
  1 level tsp low-sodium baking powder
  1 tsp natural vanilla essence

Pre-heat the oven to 350°F/180°C/gas mark 4. Lightly oil a baking sheet. Dice the dried apricots, place them in a small saucepan and just cover with water. Bring to the boil and simmer very gently for 30 minutes. Add a little more water if necessary to prevent them drying out. Mix the dry ingredients together.

Once the apricots are cooked, purée them with a hand blender, adding a little more water if necessary to obtain a thick, smooth purée. Stir in the vanilla essence, then mix into the dry ingredients. Incorporate thoroughly to achieve a thick, stiff paste. Roll the paste into two long sausage shapes. Divide each roll into 10 segments. Roll each segment into a ball with your hands, press your hands together to flatten it, and place it on the baking sheet. Bake in the pre-heated oven for 20 minutes.

The cookies become stale after 24 hours, but can be restored by gently warming under the grill (broiler).

Miscellaneous recipes

Basic French dressing (vinaigrette)

Ingredients
¼ pint/150 ml extra virgin olive oil
2 fl oz/55 ml wine or cider vinegar
½ tsp salt substitute
pinch mixed dried herbs
½ tsp French mustard (optional)
ground black pepper to taste

Whisk the ingredients together until thick and store refrigerated in a screw-top jar. Shake vigorously before use.

Tofu mayonnaise

Ingredients
½ packet soft silken tofu
1 tsp lemon juice
2 fl oz/55 ml extra virgin olive oil
salt substitute
ground black pepper

Liquidise the first two ingredients, then whizz in the olive oil a little at a time. Stir in the salt substitute and ground black pepper.

Variation
Before liquidising, you could also flavour this recipe with a teaspoon of mustard powder or a small sliver of raw garlic.

Date purée

Date purée is used for sweetening or can be mixed with soya cream for a delicious accompaniment to desserts. Put a generous handful of stoned dates in a small, heavy-bottomed saucepan (ideally enamelled cast iron) and just cover with water. Bring to the boil then simmer very gently with the lid on for about 10 minutes or until soft and mushy. The dates should have absorbed most of the water. If any remains, fast boil it away until there is no more than a tablespoon or two of liquid left in the pan. Remove the pan from the heat and purée the dates with a hand blender.

Home-made soya yoghurt

No special equipment is needed, but if you do have a yoghurt maker it will work just as well with soya milk as with cow's milk. Otherwise, use a bowl with a well-fitting lid or a wide-necked Thermos flask. Make sure everything is sterilised before use, as any bacteria on the utensils will compete with the yoghurt-making bacteria and the results will be disappointing.

Ingredients

17 fl oz / ½ litre unsweetened soya milk

2 tbsp starter culture (either your own previously made soya yoghurt, or a commercial brand such as Sojasun)

Boil the soya milk, then pour into a clean bowl, Thermos flask or yoghurt maker. Allow to cool to blood heat (this will take around half an hour). If you have a yoghurt or cooking thermometer, the temperature should be about 98°F/37°C; if not, a clean finger dipped into the milk works just as well – it should feel 'comfortable' at blood heat.

Stir the soya yoghurt starter into the milk and whisk briefly. If using the yoghurt maker, follow the manufacturer's instructions. Otherwise, if using a bowl, place the lid firmly on top and wrap securely in a towel or tea cosy to retain the heat. Place in a warm part of the kitchen such as above the fridge or in a warm airing cupboard for 12 hours. If using a Thermos flask, simply tighten the screw top and leave for 12 hours.

Finally, empty into a lidded container and keep refrigerated until use.

The consistency of home-made soya yoghurt is variable. Sometimes it can be quite runny and other times well set. If yours turns out to be runny, beat it well with a clean spoon (keeping it in the receptacle you made it in), replace the lid and put it in the fridge. After a few hours it should have thickened a little. Runny yoghurt can still be used for soups, casseroles and muesli.

Spelt pastry (pie crust)

Ingredients
    4 oz/115 g spelt flour
    2 oz/55 g full-fat soya flour
    approx 3½ fl oz/100 ml cold water

Sift the spelt flour into a mixing bowl. Add the soya flour and mix well with a fork. Gradually, add enough cold water to make a firm dough. Knead very lightly and place in a polythene bag. Store in the fridge for at least 1 hour. Roll out on a floured board and use as required.

Flatbread
This is a versatile chappati-type bread that can be used as a pizza base, an accompaniment to curry, a base for open sandwiches or split open and stuffed like pitta bread with a variety of fillings.

Ingredients to make approximately 9 flatbreads
    10 oz/275 g spelt flour
    2 tbsp soya yoghurt (*see recipe, p.269*)
    a few drops of warm water

Pre-heat a dry griddle pan or cast iron frying pan on a moderate heat for about 2 minutes (do not oil the pan). Add the yoghurt and enough warm water to the flour and mix to a soft, pliable dough. Turn out on to a well-floured board and knead lightly, adding more flour if necessary to prevent sticking. Break off egg-sized pieces of dough, and using more flour, roll out into rounds measuring about 6 inches / 15 cm in diameter and ¼ inch / ½ cm thick. Add more flour to the board as necessary and dust each round with a little flour before cooking.

When the pan is hot, place a round of dough on it and cook for 1½–2 minutes on each side or until small brown spots appear. To complete the cooking, place the flatbreads in a toaster or under a pre-heated grill. The breads should puff up. Don't leave them to cook for too long at this stage or they will become hard. Serve immediately.

The dough will keep overnight if covered and stored in the fridge. It does tend to become stickier with keeping, so extra flour should be kneaded in before rolling out.

To freeze
Allow the breads to cool after cooking on the griddle pan and omit the toasting / grilling stage. Place in polythene freezer bags before freezing. To use, simply toast or grill the breads from frozen.

Variations
Make as above to the rolling-out stage. Brush one side of each dough round with soya milk or water. Sprinkle generously with any combination of sesame seeds, sunflower seeds and linseeds, and press the seeds into the dough with the palm of your hand or the rolling pin. Cook as above.

Brown rice

Wash thoroughly, then pre-soak overnight in twice its volume of filtered water. Strain, place in a saucepan and cover generously with fresh water. Bring to the boil then cover tightly and simmer on the lowest possible heat for 20–25 minutes. Drain the rice in a sieve then return to the pan and leave covered away from the heat for 5 minutes, after which it is ready to serve.

Once cold, brown rice can be spread out on an oiled baking tray, frozen, then crumbled into grains and bagged for the freezer.

Cooking dried beans and peas

This includes haricot, kidney, borlotti or flageoli beans, black-eyed beans, butter beans (lima beans), chickpeas, marrowfat peas and split peas.

These should be soaked in water before use. Cover with four times their volume in boiling filtered water and leave overnight.

Throw away the soaking water, place the beans, just covered with fresh water, in a pressure cooker, bring to full steam, and cook for 3–10 minutes, depending on size. Pressure-cooking breaks down the poisonous lectins found in raw beans. If you do not use a pressure cooker, boil them fast for at least 10 minutes before simmering or slow-cooking. Small beans such as mung and aduki beans probably do not need pressure cooking. But conventional boiling may take up to two hours to soften some beans, depending on age and size.

To freeze, allow to cool and follow the same procedure as for frozen brown rice.

Drinks

It is best to drink home-made juices the same day you make them.

Home-made apple, celery, parsley and radish juice

Ingredients to make 1 serving
   1 large sweet apple, unpeeled and organically grown if possible
   2 sticks celery
   1 bunch parsley
   2 inch/5 cm segment of white mooli (icicle) radish
   a small piece of lemon (optional, though you may find that it
      helps the flavour), including peel

Wash the ingredients, cut them into chunks and put them through a juice extractor. Stir and leave to stand for 20 minutes to break down the peppery taste of the radish before drinking.

Beetroot, celery and lemon juice

Combine equal quantities of bottled beetroot juice and home-made celery juice (made from fresh celery with a juice extractor). Flavour with a little fresh lemon juice to taste. If you juice your own raw beetroot, it will be very strong and only a little is required. It must be left to stand for 20 minutes before drinking or else it will have a very peppery taste.

Home-made broccoli stem and sharp apple juice

Broccoli juice is very sweet, which is why it is good mixed with a fairly sharp apple juice. Simply cut the broccoli stems and apples into chunks and feed into your juice extractor in the proportions you prefer. You may need to experiment a little. If necessary, add a little lemon juice to disguise the broccoli flavour.

Carrot and orange juice

This is a lovely sweet combination. Simply mix half carrot juice and half orange juice together. If you do not have a juice extractor, use commercial juices and use your liquidiser to whizz in a piece of orange peel with the pith still attached.

Flavonoid-rich orange juice

Liquidise a piece of fresh orange with pith and peel into a glass of normal orange juice. This will contain a far larger quantity of flavonoids than you could get in a flavonoid supplement pill!

Home-made clover tea

Clover blossoms grow almost anywhere there is long grass. Pick them in a clean spot (not the roadside, which may be contaminated with dust from car exhausts) and dry them in the sun to bring out the coumarin, then steep them in boiling water for 5 minutes, strain and drink the liquid. You could also add some grated ginger, chamomile, orange or lemon zest. Some specialist herbal suppliers sell dried clover flowers.

Broad bean tea

Save the outer green pods from fresh broad beans and dry them in the oven overnight on its lowest possible setting. Crush the pods or briefly whizz in a food processor and keep in a tightly lidded container.

To make broad bean tea, put 2 tsp broad bean pod pieces in a mug and pour over ½ pint/275 ml of boiling water and leave to infuse for 5 minutes before drinking. This tea can also be enhanced with spices such as cloves, cinnamon, ginger and cardamom.

Almond milk

This delicious drink is made by soaking a large handful of blanched almonds in 1 pint/570 ml water overnight in the goblet of your liquidiser. In the morning whizz them together until the almonds have turned into a fine pulp and strain the milk through a fine sieve. The result is naturally sweet and excellent for drinking, while the pulp can be added to rice pudding.

Variation

Try the same method with other nuts, such as Brazils and cashews.

Home-made ginger tea with lemon zest

Pour a cupful of boiling water on to a teaspoon of grated fresh ginger and a teaspoon of fresh lemon zest shreds. Leave to infuse for 5 minutes, then strain and drink. This is an excellent drink if you feel a cold coming on, or to settle your stomach if you have a tummy upset.

Useful Addresses

Linda Lazarides' website

With internet community, details of my other publications and much useful information on all aspects of nutritional therapy. You can also subscribe to my occasional newsletters with updates on the Waterfall Diet and other health issues.

www.health-diets.net

International Society for Orthomolecular Medicine

Find doctors all over the world who use vitamin therapy.

www.orthomed.org/isom/isom.html

Life Extension Foundation

International suppliers of health supplements.

www.lef.org

Lymphoedema website

Much useful information, including suppliers of coumarin in different countries and Casley-Smith-trained massage therapists.

www.lymphoedema.org.au

The Vegan Society

Can provide scientific information written by qualified state-registered dieticians on the health and safety of diets free of dairy and other animal produce.

Donald Watson House, 21 Hylton Street, Hockley, Birmingham B18 6HJ, United Kingdom. Tel: +44 (0)121 523 1730. E-mail: info@vegansociety.com

www.vegansociety.com

United Kingdom

Abel & Cole Limited

Organic vegetables, fruit, meat etc. delivered to your door. The emphasis is on British produce.

16 Waterside Way, Plough Lane, Wimbledon, London SW17 0HB.

Tel: 08452 626364. E-mail: organics@abelandcole.co.uk

www.abelandcole.co.uk

Ardovries Shearway Ltd

Suppliers of frozen blueberries, Black Forest fruits and frozen organic vegetables to supermarkets. Phone to find stockists.

WaySearch, Smarden Road, Headcorn, Kent, TN27 9TA.

Tel: 01622 891 199

Breakspear Hospital for Allergy and Environmental Medicine

Hertfordshire House, Wood Lane, Hemel Hempstead, Herts., HP2 4FD, UK. Tel: 01442 261333. E-mail: info@breakspearmedical.com

www.breakspearmedical.com

The British Association for Nutritional Therapy

Send large SAE and £2 for a list of practitioners.

27 Old Gloucester St, London WC1N 3XX. Tel: 08706 061284.

E-mail: theadministrator@bant.org.uk

www.bant.org.uk

The British Society for Ecological Medicine

Doctors specialising in nutritional medicine and the treatment of allergies and food intolerances.

c/o New Medicine Group, PO Box 3AP, London W1A 3AP.

Tel: 0207 100 7090. E-mail: info@ecomed.org.uk

www.ecomed.org.uk

Clearspring Ltd

Health and macrobiotic foods, rice milk, seaweed products. Their excellent products are now stocked in most larger supermarkets, including Sainsbury's, Tesco, Waitrose and Morrisons, and are also available by mail order. See their website

for distributors in other European countries, the Middle East and the Far East.
Unit 19A Acton Park Estate, London W3 7QE.
Tel: 020 8749 1781. E-mail: mailorder@clearspring.co.uk
www.clearspring.co.uk

BEAT (Beating Eating Disorders)

Help and guidance for those with anorexia, bulimia and other eating disorders.
103 Prince of Wales Road, Norwich, Norfolk, NR1 1DW. Tel: 0300 1233355.
www.b-eat.co.uk

The Healthy House

House paints, etc., for people with allergic illness and chemical sensitivities.
The Old Co-op, Lower Street, Ruscombe, Stroud, Gloucestershire, GL6 6BU.
Tel: 01453 752216. E-mail: info@healthy-house.co.uk
www.healthy-house.co.uk

The Nutri Centre

Mail order suppliers of all available food supplements in UK.
Unit 3, Kendal Court, Kendal Avenue, London W3 0RU. Tel: 0845 602 6744.
E-mail: admin@nutricentre.com
www.nutricentre.com

Riverford Organic Vegetables Limited

Award-winning fresh organic fruit, salads, vegetables, herbs, meat, wine,
beer, etc. delivered to your door.
Wash Barn, Buckfastleigh, Devon, TQ11 0JU. Tel: 0845 600 2311.
www.riverford.co.uk

The Soil Association

The UK's leading campaigning and certification organisation for organic
food and farming.
South Plaza, Marlborough Street, Bristol, BS1 3NX. Tel: 0117 314 5000.
www.soilassociation.org

Suppliers of gluten-free foods

Clearspring, www.clearspring.co.uk
Doves Organic, www.dovesfarm.co.uk
Eat Natural, www.eatnatural.co.uk

Health Link UK, www.healthlinkuk.com
Nature's Path, www.naturespath.com
Orgran, www.orgran.com
Real Foods, www.realfoods.co.uk
Virginia Harvest, www.virginiafoods.net

United States

The American Academy of Environmental Medicine
Register of practitioners of environmental and nutritional medicine.
6505 E. Central Avenue, #296, Wichita, KS 67206. Tel: (316) 684-5500.
E-mail: administrator@aaemonline.org
www.aaem.com

The American Association of Naturopathic Physicians
Register of practitioners of naturopathic medicine.
4435 Wisconsin Avenue, NW, Suite 403, Washington, DC 20016.
Tel: (202) 237 8150; (866) 538 2267 (toll-free from the US).
www.naturopathic.org

The American College of Advancement in Medicine
Register of practitioners.
8001 Irvine Center Drive, Suite 825, Irvine, CA 92618.
Tel: (949) 309 3520. Email: infoe@acam.org
www.acam.org

The American Environmental Health Foundation
Organisation for the recognition and appropriate treatment of environmental
illness. Books and publications available. Founded by Dr William Rea.
8345 Walnut Hill Lane, Suite 25, Dallas, TX 75231.
Tel: (214) 361 9515; (800) 428 2343. E-mail: aehf@aehf.com
www.aehf.com

Genova Diagnostics
Can put you in touch with practitioners who can arrange liver function tests
for you.
63 Zillicoa Street, Asheville, NC 28801. Tel: (800) 522 4762.
www.GDX.net

Suppliers of gluten-free foods
Bakery on Main, www.bakeryonmain.com
The Better Health Store, www.thebetterhealthstore.com
Bob's Red Mill, www.bobsredmill.com
Gluten Free Mall, www.glutenfreemall.com
Nature's Path, www.naturespath.com
U.S. Mills (Erewhon), www.usmillsllc.com

Australia

The Australasian College of Nutritional and Environmental Medicine
Referral service for all conventionally trained GPs and specialists who are
interested in a wider and more natural approach to illness.
10/23–25 Melrose Street, Sandringham, Victoria 3191. Tel: (03) 9597 0363. E-
mail: mail@acnem.org
www.acnem.org

The Australian Natural Therapists' Association
PO Box 657, Maroochydore BC Qld 4558. Free-call: 1800 817 577.
www.australiannaturaltherapistsassociation.com.au

The Natural Health Society of Australia
Not-for profit organisation. Information on practitioners and products.
Skiptons Arcade, Suite 28, 541 High Street, Penrith NSW 2750.
Tel: (02) 4721 5068. E-mail: info@health.org.au
http://health.org.au

Suppliers of gluten-free foods
Energy Products, www.energyproducts.com.au
Orgran, www.orgran.com

Canada

The Society for Orthomolecular Medicine
E-mail: centre@orthomed.org to request a list of doctors and practitioners
in your province who use vitamin therapy.
www.orthomed.org

New Zealand

The NZ Charter of Health Practitioners
The New Zealand Charter of Health Practitioners Incorporated, 2 Airborne Road, Albany, North Shore Auckland. Tel: (09) 414–5501.
www.healthcharter.org.nz

The NZ Society of Naturopaths
PO Box 90–170, Victoria Street West, Auckland 1142
www.naturopath.org.nz

The Soil & Health Association of New Zealand
Information on products, therapies, practitioners. Publications available.
PO Box 36170, Northcote, Auckland. Tel: (09) 419 4536.
www.organicnz.org

Resources for lymphoedema

> Do not take any of these products (including those which require no prescription) unless your doctor has specifically diagnosed you with lymphoedema.

Suppliers of coumarin and flavonoid products for lymphoedema
Information from www.lymphoedema.org.au

Coumarin for lymphoedema
All countries except USA and Canada
Lympedim® (Coumarin) 200 mg. tablets. Pharm Products, Private Ltd., 'Vijai', Medical College Rd, Thanjavur 613007, Tamil Nadu, India. Tel: 91+ (4362) 239176. Fax: 91+ (4362) 231650. E-mail: pplm@dataone.in
Chennai office: Tel: 91+(44) 6213496. Fax: 91+(44) 6222415.
E-mail: ppplm@vsnl.com
www.pharmproducts.com
Ask your doctor for a prescription for two of these tablets per day. Give these contact details to your pharmacist.

USA and Canada

In the USA coumarin is only authorised for research use. It is available (by prescription only) from compounding pharmacists:

Barry Smith, Medical-Dental Pharmacy, 689 E. Nees, Fresno, California 93720, USA. Tel: (559) 439-1190, (800) 794-2832. Fax: (559) 439-1655.

E-mail: mdpii@aol.com

Oral (200 or 400 mg delayed-release capsules), 10 per cent ointment and 10 per cent powder are all available from the above. Your doctor can consult this pharmacist about the recommended dosages.

Flavonoids for lymphoedema

Lympaction® Poppy Lane Skin Care and Lymphoedema Clinic, 139 Hollywood Drive, Lansvale NSW 2166, Australia.

Tel: (02) 9723 5402. Fax: (02) 9726 3322. E-mail: julietgeorge@lymph.com.au

www.lymph.com.au

Lympaction® is an oral mixture of rutin and other flavonoids taken as 1½ tsp per day in a glass of water. The flavour is pleasant. This is much less expensive than many other listed products and does not need a doctor's pre-scription. Most countries will allow individuals to import this product for their own personal use.

Paroven® (Venoruton®, Relvène® from Zyma, CH-1260, Nyon, Switzerland) is available through your pharmacist in most countries of the world, but not the USA. It comes as capsules of 100, 250 or (in some countries) 500 or 1,000 mg. The minimum effective dose for lymphoedema is 3,000 mg/day (6,000 is often better). Often no prescription is necessary.

Index

How did you get on with the Waterfall Diet?

If we are to bring about any changes in the way weight problems are treated in the healthcare system, research is essential. The best way to stimulate interest for the funding of such research is to show doctors and dieticians a wealth of case histories.

If you have read this book and tried the Waterfall Diet, your feedback would be very much appreciated. To help others, could I ask you to complete the following questionnaire? If you do not want to cut it out of the book, please feel free to write your answers on a separate piece of paper.

Waterfall Diet Questionnaire

1. How much did you weigh before starting the Waterfall Diet?

   _____

2. How much do you weigh now?_____

3. Were you on a calorie-controlled diet before beginning the Waterfall Diet? YES/NO
   If so, how many calories per day? _____

4. How long did you spend on Phase I of the Waterfall Diet?

   _____

5. Did you complete Phase II of the Waterfall Diet? YES/NO
6. How easy did you find the Waterfall Diet (please tick as appropriate)?
   ☐ Impossible, I gave up after _____ days because

   _____

   _____

   _____

☐ Very difficult, but I was able to persevere.
☐ Difficult, but becoming easier as I got used to it.
☐ No more difficult than other diets I have tried.
☐ Relatively easy compared with other diets I have tried.
☐ Very easy.

7. How successful have you found the Waterfall Diet compared with a normal calorie-controlled diet (please tick as appropriate)?
☐ Much more successful.
☐ About the same.
☐ Less successful.
☐ Not effective at all.

8. What type of fluid retention do the questionnaires suggest you had (please tick as appropriate)?
☐ Allergic.
☐ Protein deficiency.
☐ Kidney stress.
☐ Prescription medicines.
☐ Internal pollution.
☐ Capillary or lymphatic problems.
☐ Vitamin or mineral deficiencies.

9. Do you think doctors and dieticians should be trained in the principles of the Waterfall Diet? YES/NO

10. Do you have any other comments about the Waterfall Diet?

_____

_____

_____

11. I agree/do not agree (delete as appropriate) that this information and my contact details can be passed on to a health writer with a view to publicising the benefits of the Waterfall Diet.

_____

Your name and contact details:

_____

_____

_____

Thank you so much for your assistance. Please send your answers to:

Linda Lazarides
BCM Waterfall
London WC1N 3XX
United Kingdom

Or fill in the on-line form at:

www.health-diets.net/water-retention/wfdiet-survey.htm

Readers are welcome to join my internet community at
www.health-diets.net/water-retention

I am available for online consultations and you can also
subscribe to my free e-mail newsletters.